The Design, Construction and Use of Removable Orthodontic Appliances

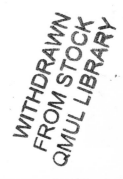

The Design, Construction and Use of Removable Orthodontic Appliances

C. Philip Adams MDS, FDS, DOrth., RCSEng., FFDRCSI

Emeritus Professor, Queens University, Belfast; Honorary Consultant, Eastern Health and Social Services Board

W. John S. Kerr MDS, DOrth., RCSEng., FDS, RCSEdin, FFDRCSI, FDS, RCPSGlas

Reader in Orthodontics, University of Glasgow; Honorary Consultant, Greater Glasgow Health Board

Butterworth–Heinemann
London   Boston   Singapore   Sydney   Toronto   Wellington

Wright
is an imprint of Butterworth–Heinemann Ltd

 PART OF REED INTERNATIONAL P.L.C.

First published 1990

© **Butterworth–Heinemann Ltd, 1990**

British Library Cataloguing in Publication Data

Adams, C. P. (Charles Philip)
   The design, construction and use of removable
   orthodontic appliances.
   1. Man. Removable orthodontic appliances
   I. Title   II. Kerr, W. John S.
   617.6430028

ISBN 0-7236-2111-X

Library of Congress Cataloging-in-Publication Data

Adams, C. Philip (Charles Philip)
   The design, construction, and use of removable
   orthodontic appliances/C. Philip Adams,
W. John S. Kerr. – [6th ed.]
      p.   cm.
   Rev. ed. of: The design and construction of
removable orthodontic appliances. 4th ed. 1970.
   Includes bibliographical references.
   Includes index.
   ISBN 0-7236-2111-X
   1. Orthodontics.   2. Dental instruments and
apparatus.   I. Kerr, W. John S.   II. Adams, C.
Philip (Charles Philip) Design and construction of
removable orthodontic appliances.   III. Title.
   [DNLM: 1. Orthodontic Appliances, Removable
   WU 400 A211d]
RK528.M4A45   1990
617.6′43′0028–dc20
DNLM/DLC   90-2586
for Library of Congress   CIP

Composition by Genesis Typesetting, Rochester, Kent
Printed and bound in Great Britain by Courier
International Ltd., Tiptree, Essex

Preface to the Sixth Edition

The continued growth of interest in the provision of orthodontic services and the expansion in the teaching of the subject at undergraduate and postgraduate levels that have taken place in recent years have together reinforced the ongoing need for a better understanding of the potential of removable orthodontic appliances. These factors have been borne in mind in the preparation of this new edition and account has been taken of the greater emphasis that is now being placed on orthodontics in undergraduate and postgraduate teaching.

The result has been a streamlining of two important parts of the book. Firstly the introduction and the second chapter dealing with basic principles and design have been revised. In the past these chapters tended to overlap and they have been rewritten in an effort to make them fulfil their intended purposes more concisely and exactly.

Secondly, the final chapter dealing with technical procedures, materials and record casts has been divided into separate Appendices so that each section can be given due emphasis, especially the first two dealing with technical procedures and clasp design and construction. The matters dealt with in these sections seem to have been not always well understood and so to have been a source of weakness in much removable appliance design, construction and use. It is hoped that by identifying these subjects more clearly, doubts and misunderstandings might be removed and the importance of good techniques and good design better appreciated.

All the material in the appendices has been rewritten more concisely to convey the essence of the subject matter and give the illustrations a more important role.

Further material has been added to the chapter on extra-oral appliances regarding ready-made headgear and the importance of safe headgear. The results of recent research on the effects of Fränkel appliances have been included and the Bionator has joined the list of functional appliances. There is a new chapter on management of the patient and the appliance.

There are many new illustrations, some to illustrate new material and others to replace existing illustrations more clearly and with greater impact.

We are greatly indebted to Professor Andrew Richardson for his encouragement in the preparation of this new edition and for kindly giving access to facilities in his department. We wish to thank Hill Mercer and Tom Slavin for the constructing appliances and clinical records and Sheena Sloan, Marlene Boe and Kay Shepherd for photographic illustrations.

We wish to make acknowledgement and express our thanks to: The European Orthodontic Society for permission to reproduce *Figures 1.1* and *5.15*; Mr G. G. T. Fletcher and Messrs John Wright & Sons Ltd, Bristol for permission to reproduce *Figures 1.4.* and *1.5*; Professor Arne Björk and Sveriges Tandläkarförbunds Förlagsförening, Stockholm for permission to include a personal communication in Chapter 8; Henry Kimpton, London for permission to include two quotations from their *Textbook of Functional Jaw Orthopaedics* by K. Häupl, W. J. Grossmann and P. Clarkson; the European Orthodontic Society for permission to reproduce a lengthy quotation from Dr Fränkel's paper from the Society's Transactions of 1966; The European Orthodontic Society for permission to reproduce the substance of a paper by C. P. Adams published in the Society's Transactions of 1969; Dr Egil P. Harvold and the C. V. Mosby Co. for permission to reproduce *Figure 8.59*; Dr T. M. Graber and the C. V. Mosby Co. for permission to to include quotations from *Orthodontics: Current Principles and Techniques*; Ortho-Care (U.K.) Ltd for permission to reproduce *Figures A1.3* and *B1.3A and B* from their publication *A Manual of Wire and Metal Forming with Universal Ultra Pliers*.

We are grateful to our wives for their continuous support and encouragement in our work and wish to thank Lucy Sayer and Anne Smith of Butterworth–Heinemann for their patience, help and guidance on the complexities of bringing this new edition to completion.

C. P. A.
W. J. S. K.

Contents

Chapter 1

Introduction

Orthodontic appliances can take a great variety of forms from baseplates bearing clasps and simple springs to complicated fixed appliances bonded to the teeth with connecting archwires secured to them. All orthodontic appliances, of whatever type, are intended to alter the pressure environment of the teeth in ways that are calculated to bring about new and better tooth arrangements and occlusal relationships. The dentition undergoes continual changes and variations of the pressures that are present in the dentofacial complex from the time when the facial structures are formed and begin to function, until old age when the teeth and alveolar structures are finally lost. The teeth are, therefore, continually moving. Natural tooth movement is rapid during the development of the occlusion, slower after maturity of the dentition and very slight as the occlusion wears down and teeth are lost, causing breaks in the continuity of the dental arches.

The capacity of the supporting structures to remodel as the teeth erupt naturally and when pressures are applied artificially makes orthodontic treatment possible. Orthodontic appliances exert the pressures required to produce tooth movements in various ways.

Types of orthodontic appliances

Removable appliances are clasped to the teeth and incorporate springs, elastics or screws which store pressure. Functional appliances redirect the pressures exerted by the masticatory muscles or the musculatures of the tongue, lips and cheeks. Multiband appliances make use of flexible archwires and added springs, both of which store pressure.

Clasped removable appliances

These are often referred to as 'fixed plates' and consist of a pressure source, supported by a baseplate which is clasped to the dental arch and serves to distribute the reaction to the force exerted over the anchorage area or base.

Springs are the commonest pressure sources and they can be of various shapes but are usually of a cantilever type or some modification of it. A cantilever spring is fixed at one end and deflected at the other within the elastic limit of the spring material. In returning to its position of rest, the spring delivers the amount of pressure required to produce the deflection.

Bands of rubber or latex of various sizes and thicknesses can be stretched between hooks attached to teeth or appliances to apply traction for the movement of single teeth or groups of teeth.

Orthodontic screw devices have left and right-hand threads at opposite ends. When the screw is turned, the segments of the baseplate at either side move apart producing pressure on the teeth to which they are attached.

Functional appliances

Functional appliances make use of the forces exerted by the muscles of the tongue, face and neck and the muscles of mastication. These muscle systems, together with the tissues connected with them, produce pressures on the tooth crowns which affect the positions of the teeth in a labiolingual direction. The muscles of mastication produce pressures between the dental arches which it is believed are important for the proper development of the masticatory face (see Figures 8.28, 8.40).

Functional appliances make use of these muscular

systems by inhibiting the ill effects of muscular malfunction which is producing an occlusal anomaly or by using the activity of one or other or of both of the muscle systems to produce beneficial changes in the arrangement of the teeth.

It is sometimes asserted that functional appliances stimulate development of the jaws and produce correction of discrepancies in dental base relationships. Statistical investigation suggests that small changes of this kind occur but such changes are usually of a small order and not clinically significant.

Fixed appliances

Fixed appliances are attached to the teeth by bands or by bonding specialized attachments directly to the teeth. Early fixed appliances employed the same mechanical principles as removable appliances with screws connecting teeth to be moved and heavy archwires bearing springs attached by solder or by welding (*Figure 1.1.*).

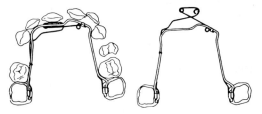

Figure 1.1 A typical labiolingual appliance consisting of molar bands with a heavy lingual arch and a fine spring to procline the right upper central incisor

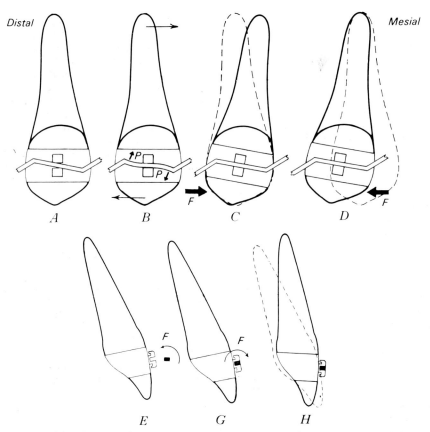

Figure 1.2 The edgewise arch; second-order bends. *A*, The passive arch crosses the bracket at an angle; *B*, the archwire is deformed in order to get it into the channel and the resulting pressures, *PP*, tend to tilt the apex mesially, the crown distally; *C*, if the crown is stabilized with a force, *F*, the main movement will take place at the apex; *D*, if the crown is assisted to move by force *F*, the main movement will take place at the crown and not at the apex; *E*, torque force applied to an incisor using the edgewise arch for labial root movement. The arch must be twisted with a force *F* to align it with the channel in the bracket and so permit insertion; *G*, the arch then exerts force *F* tipping the apex of the tooth labially. The amount of pressure exerted on the labial plate of bone is difficult to measure clinically; *H*, movement produced by torque force

The development of the multiband appliance with a continuous archwire connecting all the teeth introduced new methods of pressure application and anchorage.

Forces are produced in multiband appliances by forming the archwire so that when it is pinned or tied into the attachments fixed to the teeth it imposes movements on any tooth or group of teeth that may be required. It is also possible to develop pressures on teeth by using a plain flat archwire and aligning the attachments on the teeth so as to generate forces when the archwire is ligatured into the channels on the attachments.

The edgewise appliance was introduced by Edward Angle (1929) as 'the latest and best in orthodontic mechanisms' after a series of developments from the ribbon arch appliance which made use of a ribbon-like arch which was laid flat against the labial surfaces of the teeth. The edgewise arch was so named because the wire was rectangular in section and lay with the smaller dimension towards the teeth. The brackets were made so that the archwire fitted accurately into the channels so ensuring accurate tooth positioning.

The edgewise arch is shaped into an ideal form and ligatured into the channels in the brackets. The dental arches are aligned in perfect arrangement and the occlusal relationship corrected by intermaxillary and extra-oral traction. Mesiodistal and labiolingual inclinations can be adjusted by second- and third-order bends which are formed by placing steps in the archwire and small twists which torque the roots labiolingually and mesiodistally. Complete control of tooth positioning can be achieved. Angle maintained that all teeth could be brought into perfect occlusion with this appliance (*Figure 1.2*).

The way in which multiband appliances are attached to the teeth breaks up the length of the archwire into short sections which act as beam springs and this makes it possible to develop high pressures if the archwire is fully seated in the brackets. One method of reducing the possibility of generating too high pressures is to use fine archwire when the pressure exerted for any given degree of deflection will be less.

The twin wire arch appliance devised by Johnson (1938) was a move towards exerting smaller pressures with fixed appliances. The Johnson twin wire arch made use of two wires of 0.25 mm thickness ligatured into simple channel attachments on the six upper and lower anterior teeth. The ends of the archwires were supported in lengths of tubing which lay in tubes attached to the first molar teeth. This appliance produces excellent alignment of the teeth of the labial segments and arch relationships can be corrected by intermaxillary traction (*Figure 1.3*).

The best known and still used light wire appliance system is that devised by Begg (1965) in which a series of archwires is used starting at 0.35 mm and increasing to 0.5 mm as tooth alignment is achieved. The attachments in this appliance permit the teeth to move freely along the archwire and to tilt and rotate, these movements being produced and controlled by adjustments of the archwire itself in the early stages of treatment when irregularities of the teeth are smoothed out and extraction sites are closed by tilting the adjacent teeth together (*Figures 1.4, 1.5*).

In the later stages a thicker, plain archwire is used and the final aligning of the teeth adjacent to extraction sites is effected by torquing the roots of the teeth with auxiliary springs. Intermaxillary traction is used to correct arch relationship antero-posteriorly but, according to the rationale of the treatment method, extra-oral traction is not required.

The straight wire appliance, devised by Andrews (1972), has some features in common with the twin wire arch in that a preformed archwire is used to which tooth alignment is made to conform by ligaturing the archwire into attachments on the teeth. Preformed straight wire arches are more sophisticated than the twin wire arch in that the straight wire lies flat and edgewise to the teeth and the attachments are made with differing degrees of inbuilt mesiodistal and labiolingual torque. By selecting and bonding appropriate attachments to the teeth, a full range of planned tooth movements can be effected by placing and ligaturing a simple, plain archwire.

Combinations of fixed and removable appliances

Figure 1.6 shows a case where slight elongation of a tooth was needed following delayed eruption due to a supernumerary tooth which was removed. A bracket is cemented to the affected central incisor and a spring is brought forward from a baseplate and activated gently in a downward direction. The patient lifts the spring into place after inserting the baseplate. Such a movement is effected carefully and progress monitored frequently.

A single tooth may be rotated or the root torqued by means of a simple spring attached to the tooth by a box, socket or tube, hooking the free end onto the bridge of a clasp on a baseplate and so avoiding the necessity of using a full multiband appliance. The patient can unhook the spring and remove the baseplate for cleaning and re-hook the spring which automatically produces activation (*see Figure 5.17*).

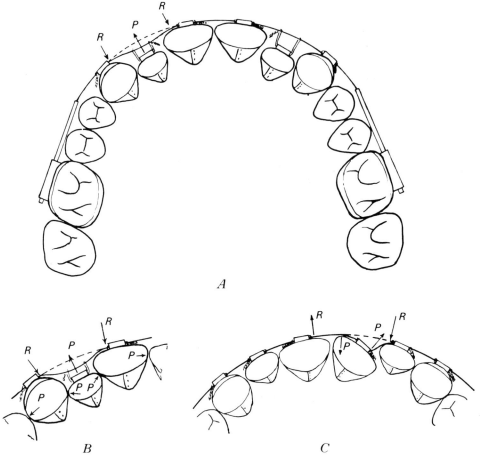

A

B   *C*

Figure 1.3 *A*, Labial movement with the twin wire arch *P*, pressure on the upper right lateral incisor; *R*, the reaction. The reaction is borne mainly by the adjoining teeth. The ligature on the left lateral incisor has not yet been tightened; *B*, when the incisors are imbricated, the full pressure, *P*, of the twin wire is not taken by the single displaced tooth. The reaction, *RR*, remains the same on the adjoining teeth, but the pressure, *P*, is dispersed against their sloping lingual surfaces, forcing them apart, and hence against the next two teeth in the row; *C*, rotation of an incisor with the twin wire arch;

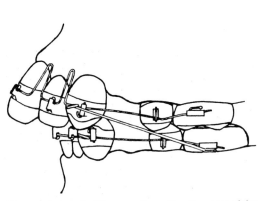

Figure 1.4. A typical Begg appliance for alignment of the anterior segments, reduction of overbite and closure of extraction sites by lingual movement of upper labial segment and mesial movement of lower molars and second premolars

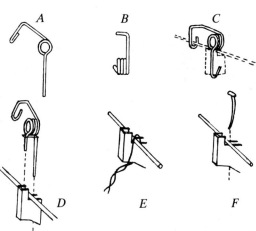

A   *B*   *C*

D   *E*   *F*

Figure 1.5. Auxiliary springs for the Begg appliance. *A–D*, A root torquing auxiliary ligature and lockpin with *E–F*, unipoint bracket

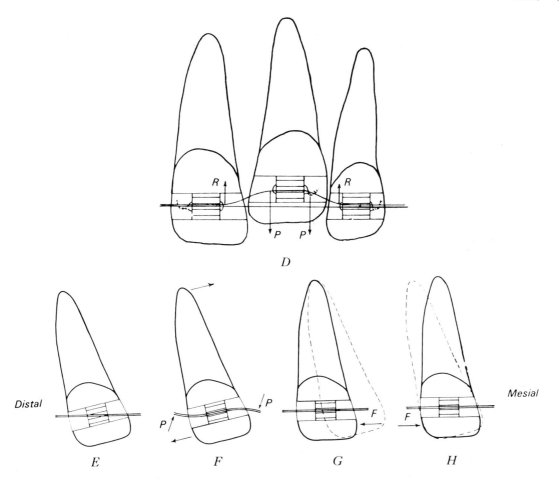

D

Distal

Mesial

E   *F*   *G*   *H*

Figure 1.3 continued *D*, elongation of a tooth with the twin wire arch. Light pressure is used, the reaction is unlikely to upset the adjoining teeth; *E*, the arch is passive; *F*, the arch must be deformed to get it into the bracket. The resulting pressures tend to move the root mesially and the crown distally; *G*, if the crown is assisted by a force, *F*, movement will be mostly at the crown; *H*, if the crown is stabilized with a force, movement will take place at the apex

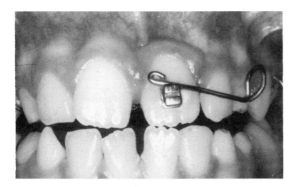

Figure 1.6. A combined fixed-removable appliance for elongation of a tooth. A spring anchored in a baseplate is brought forward to lie on the attachment and very gently activated downwards. The loop renders the spring flexible and the end of the spring is recurved into a smooth loop

Conclusions

Removable appliances have many advantages; they exert minimal interference with dentoalveolar growth, and are particularly useful for treatment during the developing stages of the dentition. Removable appliance treatment, taking place at earlier ages, is attractive as it offers early completion dates and little inconvenience during socially and educationally busy years for the growing child.

The success of removable appliances depends on good design and attention to detail. Collaboration between the user of an appliance (the orthodontist) and the producer (the technician) must be close. Removable appliances must be well designed and accurately constructed to the specification of the orthodontist who, if necessary, must be able to construct an appliance himself exactly as he wants it.

Chapter 2

The design of removable appliances

The design of a removable appliance or fixed plate entails the pressure source to be used and its effects in producing the desired tooth movement, the dispersal of the reaction of the force to the anchorage and the effects on the anchorage, the clasping requirements of the appliance and the layout of the baseplate.

These factors will arise in the order mentioned but as the design evolves, one or other factor may be reconsidered until the most satisfactory design is decided on.

Pressure sources

Springs

The most suitable material for orthodontic springs is stainless steel wire containing 18% nickel and 8% chromium. This is known as 18/8 stainless steel and it combines elasticity and malleability in excellent proportions and is tasteless and immune to corrosion by the oral secretions.

The most generally useful spring for removable appliances is the cantilever spring. Experience and familiarity with the manipulation of orthodontic wires conveys a good sense of the forces exerted by wires of different thickness and lengths. In scientific terms, the connection between the length, thickness and amount of deflection of a cantilever spring of round section is expressed by the formula

$$D \propto PL^3/T^4$$

where D is the amount of deflection, P the amount of pressure, L the length of the spring and T the thickness (*Figure 2.1*).

This means that for a given cantilever spring, deflection will be double when pressure is doubled,

deflection will increase by eight times if the length of the spring is doubled and 16 times if the thickness of the wire is halved. It is important to understand how the dimensions of a wire theoretically affect the physical properties of a spring although it will be found that in practice, the design and construction of springs becomes fairly standardized for the various movement needs that arise in treatment.

When designing a spring for a particular tooth movement, the requirements are to ensure that the spring will act over the distance and in the direction needed to move the tooth that is being treated, that the spring will exert a suitable pressure to produce tooth movement and that the spring will at the same time be mechanically strong enough to withstand the interferences that occur in the mouth in eating and speaking and during cleaning after meals.

Planning the design and layout of a spring entails selecting a point of attachment so that the free end sweeps along the intended line of movement of the tooth; further details are to ensure an optimum combination of length, number of coils, thickness, shape of the spring and provision for guarding and guiding the spring over its range of activity. If these features are well conceived, the resulting appliance will be comfortable to wear, sure in action, trouble-free and easy for the patient to insert, remove and keep clean.

The amount of deflection produced by a number of springs commonly used on removable appliances is shown in *Table 2.1*. The deflections are those produced by a pressure of 20 g for comparison of the performance of springs of differing length, thickness and size and number of coils. It should be borne in mind that as the springs return to their positions of rest the pressures they exert fall to zero, and that as these springs will be being used on teeth larger than the smallest single-rooted tooth, in practice the

Table 2.1 Table of pressures of springs

Spring type	Length (mm)	Thickness (mm)	No. of coils	Inner diameter of coils (mm)	Deflection for 20 g pressure (mm)
Apron	12	0.3	4	1.0	9.0
Finger	18	0.5	1	2.5	3.0
Self-supporting	10	0.7	1	3.5	0.3
	15	0.7	1	4.0	0.6

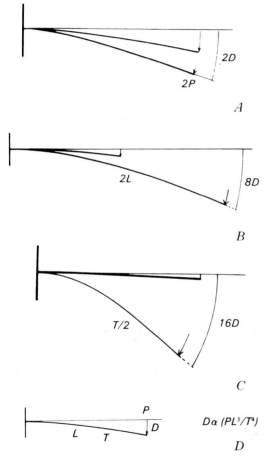

Figure 2.1 A cantilever spring is fixed at one end and free to move at the other which deflects under pressure and delivers a gradually diminishing pressure in returning to its original form; *A*, the degree of pressure is proportional to the amount of deflection produced; *B*, if the length of the spring is doubled, the degree of deflection becomes eight times as great for the same amount of pressure; *C*, if the thickness of the spring is reduced to one-half, the amount of deflection becomes 16 times as great for the same amount of pressure; *D*, deflection, pressure length and thickness are related by the formula at the right of the illustration

amounts of deflection permissible will be somewhat larger than those shown in the table.

Any piece of stainless steel wire of any length or thickness can be used as a spring as long as the amount of pressure exerted on a tooth is not excessive. From the practical point of view the length and thickness of a spring must be decided with regard to the space available for it, and while in protected situations slimmer springs with longer ranges of action can be designed, in exposed positions shorter, thicker springs need to be used and the correspondingly short ranges of action have to be accepted. A representative selection of cantilever springs is shown in *Figure 2.2*.

The thinnest springs of 0.35 mm thickness, such as apron springs, need to be wound on heavy supports and the free ends recurved and wrapped round the supports; slightly thicker springs of 0.5 mm wire used as finger springs may be left with a free end but need to be guarded and guided to ensure that their action is confined to one plane; thick springs of 0.7 mm or more can support themselves and are not displaced by pressures of the tongue or lips. Their range of action is still enough to make them active over a four-week period and the judicious use of coils gives extra flexibility in the direction of their action.

The most effective spring is a finger spring with a coil at the point of attachment, the free end moving in a well defined arc. The direction of action of the spring can be seen and the point of application to the tooth adjusted as required. A useful variation of the cantilever spring is the double cantilever where a second limb is formed with a second coil. This spring can be used to move two or more teeth in the same direction over equal distances as when proclining two or more upper incisor teeth (*Figure 2.3*) (*see also Figure 3.13*).

Miniaturization of the double cantilever spring for use on a single tooth is not satisfactory as the spring becomes little more than a crumpled piece of wire without a positive line of action and is difficult to keep in contact with the tooth surface. For the movement of a single tooth a single cantilever spring is the best arrangement as such a spring can be seen

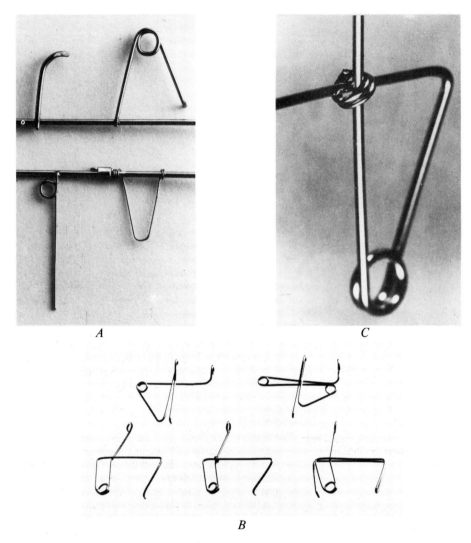

Figure 2.2 *A*, A representative group of springs fixed to a heavy support. Top row, a spring of 0.9 mm wire and a buccal canine retraction spring of 0.7 mm wire. Bottom row, a finger spring of 0.5 mm wire with one coil and an apron spring of 0.3 mm wire wound on the heavy supporting archwire; *B*, a group of cantilever springs with guards. Upper row, a single and a double cantilever spring with a guard to keep the spring applied to the tooth. Bottom row, a single cantilever spring for retraction of teeth in the buccal segments. Left, a plain spring and guard; centre, a spring with a wire link holding the spring to the guard; right, a spring with a double guide to prevent distortion of the spring by the patient; *C*, detail of a link wound round the guard and a guide wire to stop the patient lifting the spring away from the guard. A link is made of 0.3 mm wire wound round twice, cut off and loosened by pushing a probe through until the link has been slightly enlarged

to act positively and can be guided onto the point of pressure on the tooth.

Finger springs must be guarded and guided with care to ensure that they work smoothly and accurately. Guards and guides for finger springs should be made of the same kind of wire which will give a smooth guiding action. The boxing of springs beneath the baseplate should be avoided if at all possible. Springs boxed in this way cannot run

smoothly and the cavity formed by the boxing is a food trap; inflammation of the gum tissue causes it to swell into the cavity. The spring inevitably becomes lifted away from the baseplate by careless handling or during adjustment and the limb and coil of the spring cause further irritation. Such an arrangement is an endless source of trouble. A spring boxed beneath a baseplate with a superimposed wire guide is also an extremely troublesome

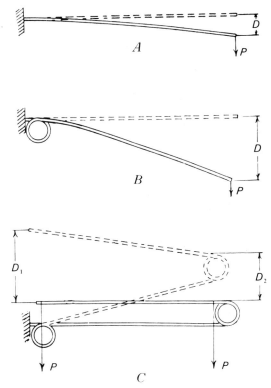

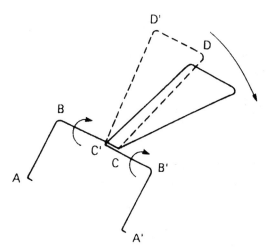

Figure 2.4 The torque spring. The ends AB and A′B′ are embedded in the baseplate. The lengths BC and B′C′ twist when the apron CD–C′D′ is deflected

Figure 2.3 *A*, A simple cantilever spring, fixed at one end and free to move at the other; *B*, cantilever spring with coil at the point of attachment to the baseplate or support; *C*, a double cantilever spring which will move two, three or four teeth an equal amount in the same direction. Pressure *P* produces deflections D, D_1 and D_2

and the sections A–B and A′–B′ are fixed in the baseplate of the appliance. The sections B–C and B′–C′ are torque bars and the sections C–D and C′–D′ make up an apron spring.

arrangement as the guide confines the spring against the baseplate making smooth action impossible and the spring is difficult to adjust. A double wire guide or a link holding the spring to the guide gives a very smooth action and an open window in the baseplate ensures cleanliness and ease of adjustment of the spring (*see Figure 2.2C*, also *Figures 3.13, 4.7* and *4.9*).

Finger springs in one form or another will be found to serve the vast majority of purposes for removable appliances. The so-called T spring is a finger spring for a situation where the addition of a coil is not feasible (*see Figure 3.25E*).

The torque spring is a special kind of finger spring where flexibility is given to a rather short and stiff acting arm by means of transverse torque limbs which derive flexibility by the twisting of two sections of wire. This spring is particularly useful where a very precise action is required on the lingual aspect of upper anterior teeth which have to be rotated. *Figure 2.4* shows diagrammatically the layout of a torque spring. The spring is symmetrical

Elastics

Elastic bands have for many years been used as a convenient means for applying pressure in orthodontic appliances. The different sizes of bands supplied by stationers, formerly used for all purposes, are now used mainly in extra-oral appliances and special elastics are available from orthodontic suppliers in numbered sizes from ⅛ inch to ⁵⁄₁₆ inch and in different thicknesses for intra-oral use (*Figure 2.5*).

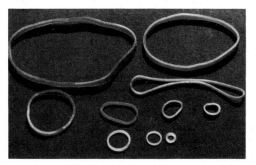

Figure 2.5 A selection of elastics. These range from the ordinary elastics available from stationers down to the specialist elastics obtained from orthodontic suppliers seen in the bottom row. The smallest of the three circular elastics is ⅛ inch in diameter

The rules for springs regarding the amount of pressure exerted on teeth apply also to elastics, and bands should be stretched sufficiently to produce the desired effect. Elastics have a considerable range of action but some kinds perish quite quickly in the oral fluids and frequent replacement is needed.

Screws

A screw consists of a rod with left and right hand threads at either end and a nut in the centre which is turned with a wrench or tommy bar. The threads turn in metal blocks which are embedded in the baseplate of the appliance which is split at right angles to the screw (*Figure 2.6*). When the screw is

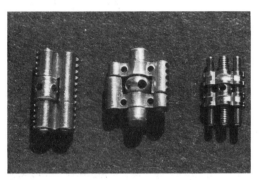

Figure 2.6 Screws for orthodontic appliances. Left, a single screw with a single guide; centre and right, double-ended screws with double guides. The screw on the right measures 11 mm in length

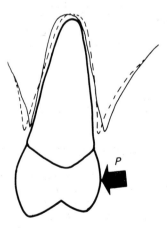

Figure 2.7 A tooth can be moved immediately by a small amount due to the elasticity of the supporting tissues. If held in the new position the alveolar bone adapts itself to the new position of the root. A pressure *P* produced by a screw plate causes movement of a tooth over a very short distance

turned, the two parts of the baseplate separate and press upon the teeth. The slight mobility of the teeth allows them to move a little and during the following weeks the bone supporting the teeth is remodelled to the new positions of the teeth. This process is repeated until the necessary tooth movement is produced (*Figure 2.7*).

Some screws incorporate a coil spring and in effect the spring is adjusted by turning the screw. The spring then exerts pressure tending to separate the two parts of the appliance.

Screw appliances are under the control of the patient who must understand how the appliance works and make adjustments to the screw at appropriate intervals.

Anchorage

Force needs to be exerted from a supporting base which serves to distribute the reaction so that it will not produce unwanted effects. The simplest way of dispersing the reaction to a force is to spread it over a large area.

The base from which a force acts is the anchorage for the force and anchorage may be arranged in removable orthodontic appliances in a number of ways.

Simple anchorage

Simple anchorage means that if a tooth is to be moved, a number of other teeth in the same arch are used to provide support for the orthodontic pressure. More teeth must be used for anchorage than are being moved orthodontically and the higher the ratio of anchorage teeth to teeth being moved, the less likelihood there is of the anchorage teeth moving as well. Unintended movement of anchor teeth is referred to as 'anchorage slippage'.

Reciprocal anchorage

If two equally sized teeth or groups of teeth are to be moved in equal and opposite directions, the force applied and the reaction are reciprocal and equal so that they cancel each other out. There is no anchorage problem in such a situation.

Stationary anchorage

When pressure is applied to the crowns of teeth that are being used as anchorage, tilting of the teeth can take place. If measures are taken to prevent such tilting occurring, the pressure applied to the teeth is distributed evenly over their whole root areas and pressure per unit of root area thereby reduced. The teeth will then be less likely to move. This arrangement is known as 'stationary' anchorage

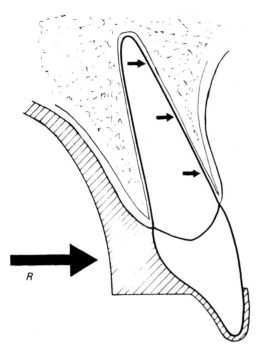

Figure 2.8 The Sved plate consists of an anterior bite-plane, the baseplate material being carried over the incisal edges of the anterior teeth. As a result, the incisors cannot incline forwards. If pressure used in the appliance has a forward reaction, *R*, this is distributed evenly along the labial wall of the incisor tooth sockets and these teeth are, as a result, more resistant to forward movement than if they were allowed to tilt. This effect is termed 'stationary anchorage'

because teeth stabilized in this way are less likely to move than teeth that are not prevented from tilting (*Figure 2.8*) (*see also Figure 7.2*).

Intermaxillary anchorage

When elastic traction is applied between the upper and lower dental arches, one whole arch acts as anchorage for the application of pressure to the other and vice versa. The elastic force applied may be acting reciprocally on both arches or one arch may be used as an anchorage base for the application of force to a segment of the opposing arch (*see Figure 7.5C*).

Extra-oral anchorage

Extra-oral anchorage may be derived from areas of the face and head outside the mouth altogether such as the back of the neck (cervical anchorage), the back of the head (occipital anchorage), or for the application of forward pressure, from the forehead and chin. All forms of extra-oral anchorage can be

regarded as stationary anchorage as the anchorage areas used do not involve possible tooth movements such as may occur in the intra-oral kinds of anchorage (*see Figure 7.9*).

Clasps

Between the maximum circumference of any tooth and the anatomical neck there are surfaces which slope inward towards the tooth axis on every side producing undercut areas (*Figures 2.9, 2.10* and *2.11*). These undercut areas are used to clasp teeth for the retention of orthodontic appliances (*Figure 2.12*).

The undercut areas on the mesial and distal aspects of the teeth begin below the contact points and are accessible quite soon after eruption of the teeth. The undercuts on the buccal and lingual aspects are much less extensive and are not accessible until the teeth are fully erupted to the anatomical neck. A clasp that makes use of the mesial and distal undercuts is the most useful as it can be used very soon after a tooth has erupted and is also more efficient than a clasp which makes use of the buccal and lingual surfaces of the teeth.

Various attempts have been made over the years to use the mesial and distal undercuts of teeth for clasping purposes and some clasps carry a wire with a small sphere on the end or a pointed arrowhead of thin wire which is lodged below the contact point between two teeth. Such clasps suffer from one disadvantage or another in either being so unobtrusive as to make removal of the appliance difficult or so obtrusive as take up excessive space and there can be difficulties in construction and adjustment.

The Adams clasp, devised in 1948, makes use of the mesial and distal undercuts and, according to Graber (1984), is the most effective and widely-used orthodontic clasp today. This clasp is strong, simple and easily constructed, it can be used on any tooth, it is neat and unobtrusive but it also makes an appliance easy to insert and remove using the bridges of the clasps. It is comfortable to wear and resistant to breakage (Hoyle, 1983; Adams, 1983; Kerr, 1983).

In planning the distribution of clasps on an appliance, it should be understood that two well-placed and well-made clasps can ensure the stability of an appliance. A line drawn from a clasp on one side of an appliance to a clasp on the other side should pass through the centre of the appliance. Two clasps placed at the distal ends of the dental arch will permit an upper appliance to drop anteriorly or a lower appliance to rise too easily. Clasps should be about the centre of the buccal segments to ensure the greatest stability of an appliance. The upper canine tooth can be clasped as

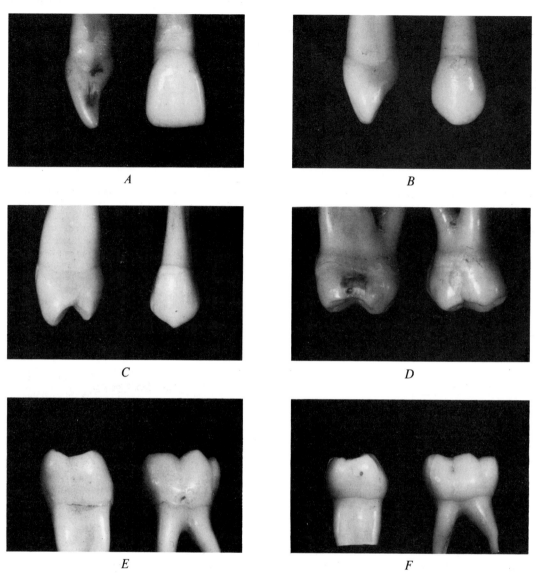

Figure 2.9 These illustrations show the mesial and the labial or buccal views of the incisor, canine, premolar and molar teeth; also the lower second deciduous molar; *A*, upper central incisor; *B*, permanent upper canine; *C*, an upper premolar; *D*, the upper first permanent molar; *E*, the lower first permanent molar; *F*, the lower second deciduous molar. These illustrations show clearly the extensive mesial and distal undercuts on all these teeth which make them suitable for orthodontic clasping

it is a strongly rooted tooth and will give additional stability to an appliance if needed, but attempts to clasp incisor teeth are to be deplored and suggest weak clasping strategy in the buccal segments.

Baseplates

Baseplates act as supports for pressure sources and distribute the reaction of these forces to the anchorage areas. Biting planes may also be incorporated in baseplates and may be aligned so that the opposing teeth bite axially, so producing a propping effect or bite on an inclined plane and producing a lateral pressure on the teeth.

Baseplates should not be too thick or larger than is necessary to distribute the reaction of the forces being used. Bite-planes should not be wider than is necessary to ensure that the opposing teeth bite squarely on them or higher than is needed to achieve

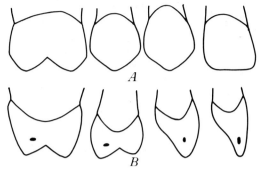

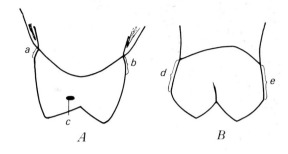

Figure 2.10 *A*, Diagram showing the extensive mesial and distal undercuts on the upper teeth from the incisors to molars which make them easy to clasp using the mesial and distal undercuts; *B*, only the premolars and molars have undercuts buccally and lingually which make them claspable but these undercuts are only available when the teeth are fully erupted

Figure 2.11 The mesial and buccal views of the upper first permanent molar comparing buccal and lingual undercuts with mesial and distal undercuts; *A*, the mesial view shows small undercuts at the buccal and lingual sides when the tooth is fully erupted, *a, b*; *B*, the undercuts mesially and distally below the contact points, *c*, can be seen from the buccal view, and are much more extensive and much more readily available for clasping at an early stage of eruption, *d, e*

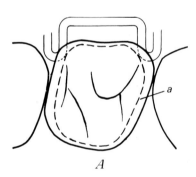

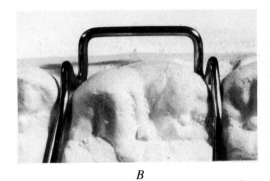

Figure 2.12 *A*, The Adams clasp which fits on a single tooth and makes use of the mesial and distal undercuts. The dotted line *a*, represents the circumference of the neck of the tooth; *B*, the clinical appearance of the Adams clasp

Figure 2.13 Baseplates should not be made unduly thick. A baseplate need not be thickened all over its area in order to embed the tags of the clasps, as in *A*. To do so fills up the mouth and interferes with speech; *p*, plaster cast, *t*, tag of clasp, *b*, baseplate material; *B*, a single thickness of wax should be used and the baseplate thickened over the tags only. This is quite as strong and much more comfortable than *A*

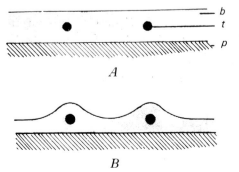

the desired bite-opening or propping effect or the required lateral pressure.

Baseplates that are too thick, extended too far in the wrong places and furnished with excessively bulky bite-planes are exceedingly uncomfortable and discouraging to wear and cause problems with eating and speaking.

A single thickness of wax is sufficient in upper baseplates and embedded wires should be retained by a thickening over the wire only and not of the entire baseplate (*Figure 2.13*).

In the upper arch trouble can arise if too much of the palate is covered by the baseplate as this will often produce nausea. The problem can be mitigated and extension of the baseplate to give maximum stability achieved if the posterior edge of the baseplate is cut forward in the centre line while at the level of the gingival margin, the baseplate is taken round the distal aspect of the last tooth (*see Figure 3.30C*). This ensures comfort in wearing the appliance and gains the maximum anchorage for the required tooth movement.

In the upper arch trouble can arise if too much of the palate is covered by the baseplate as this will often produce nausea. The problem can be mitigated and extension of the baseplate to give maximum stability achieved if the posterior edge of the baseplate is cut forward in the centre line while at the level of the gingival margin, the baseplate is taken round the distal aspect of the last tooth (*see Figure 3.30C*). This ensures comfort in wearing the appliance and gains the maximum anchorage for the required tooth movement.

To ensure that the baseplate can be inserted and removed easily it should be trimmed away from the outer side which lies against the gum tissue but not from below as this makes the baseplate too shallow. The problem can also be solved by blocking out the undercut on the plaster model before constructing the appliance. An appliance made in this way can be inserted and removed from the mouth without difficulty (*Figure 2.14*).

As with upper appliances, the disposition of clasps should ensure maximum stability (*see Figure 3.20E*). Clasping only the most distal teeth will allow an appliance to lift anteriorly too easily.

Pressure adjustment with removable orthodontic appliances

The amount of pressure exerted on a tooth has to be considered as the pressure being applied per unit of root area. Root area varies between larger and smaller teeth. It was suggested by Schwarz (1932) that a pressure of 20 g per square centimetre of root area was suitable for producing tooth movement and more recently there have been numerous investi-

gations into the effects on the periodontal tissues and tooth roots when teeth are subjected to experimental and treatment pressures in human subjects and in animals. Reitan (1985) gives a very full account of his own and others' work in this field.

There are many problems in determining exactly how the pressure on a tooth crown is finally realized at each point on a tooth root and in turn exerted at each corresponding point on the supporting tissues. In addition to the actual amount of pressure that is being exerted, factors which complicate the determination of the amount of pressure that any particular point in the periodontal tissues is being subjected to are whether the tooth is being allowed to incline or is being compelled to move in a bodily manner, the size and number of roots and hence the surface area over which the pressure is being exerted. A further factor is that the configuration of the lamina dura of the tooth socket may cause differences in the thickness of the periodontal ligament which may produce localized spots of higher pressure.

Well-conducted orthodontic treatment aims to produce 'physiological' tooth movement, that is movement associated with the normal processes of resorption and deposition of bone, so changing tooth position. When bone is removed in this way, the process is referred to as direct resorption. Investigation has shown, however, that orthodontic movement often produces hyalinization of the periodontal ligament on the side of the tooth root where pressure is exerted on the supporting structures. In hyalinized periodontal membrane, blood vessels and cells have disappeared and the tissue looks structureless and glassy. Hyalinization delays bone resorption and direct tooth movement cannot commence until the hyalinized tissue returns to normal. If the pressure is maintained, in due course undermining or secondary bone resorption in the subjacent bone takes place, relieving pressure on the hyalinized area and permitting tooth movement.

Hyalinization results from the use of high pressures in attempting to move teeth and the appearance of hyalinization when low pressures have been used appears inconsistent. Even if low pressures are used, however, irregularities in the lamina dura may produce areas against which the periodontal ligament is compressed producing spots of higher pressure which give rise to hyalinization, the effect of which is again to delay the commencement of tooth movement.

The amount of hyalinization produced is related to the amount of pressure so that there can be stages of semi-hyalinization as the structural changes progress and cells and capillaries shrink, nuclei disappear and fibre structure disintegrates and becomes confluent with the surrounding ground substance. All these processes can take place to a greater or lesser degree.

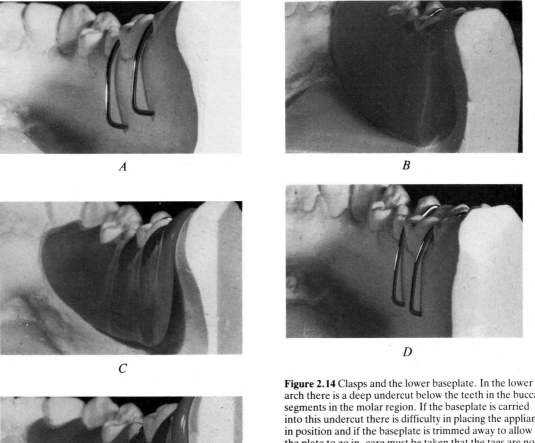

A

B

C

D

E

Figure 2.14 Clasps and the lower baseplate. In the lower arch there is a deep undercut below the teeth in the buccal segments in the molar region. If the baseplate is carried into this undercut there is difficulty in placing the appliance in position and if the baseplate is trimmed away to allow the plate to go in, care must be taken that the tags are not damaged by such trimming. To avoid this possibility, *A*, the tags of clasps may be taken down vertically and the ends turned in to touch the plaster cast; *B*, the baseplate is waxed up to cover the tags; *C*, the baseplate is trimmed away from the side towards the alveolar process so that the appliance can be inserted and the depth of the baseplate is not reduced. Alternatively, *D*, the undercut can be plastered out on the dental cast first of all and the tags of clasps made in the normal way and embedded in the baseplate as shown in *E*

The mode of force application

Ideally it would be hoped that orthodontic pressure would produce direct resorption of the bone surface without the appearance of hyalinization but such a result could only be expected under carefully controlled experimental conditions. Even if care is taken in applying orthodontic pressures to teeth, it is probable that due to the variations in the actual pressures being exerted along any root length and irregularities in the contours of the lamina dura of tooth sockets, it would be unrealistic to expect that

hyalinization would not occur at some points and if high pressures are being used, larger areas of hyalinization must occur. Vagaries in tooth movements without apparent reason may only be explicable in terms of hyalinization of the periodontal structures of the affected teeth.

Force may be exerted on a tooth continuously, intermittently or in an interrupted manner. Some writers assume that intermittent and interrupted forces are the same but Reitan (1985) regards an interrupted force as one that is exerted continuously until tooth movement is complete, as in multiband appliances where movement is effected quite quickly over a short distance and a resting period ensues until a further adjustment is made. The rigid screw type of removable appliance will operate in the same way.

An intermittent force is one that is applied and relaxed over the period between adjustments, as occurs with a removable appliance which uses a flexible and easily-adjusted spring and is taken out from time to time by the patient, and also with functional appliances which act intermittently as muscular activity energizes the appliance.

It is probable that the only example of continuous force in an orthodontic appliance is a fixed appliance with a really flexible spring attached to it and acting over the full distance of the proposed tooth movement as in the now unused labiolingual appliance. It seems unlikely that a truly continuous pressure can be developed in orthodontic treatment and that the forces that are mostly applied are either interrupted or intermittent, each of these producing slightly different effects.

A firm, interrupted force over a short distance as with a continuous archwire or screw type of appliance will produce hyalinization but the resting period between adjustments will allow secondary bone resorption and remodelling to take place. Reitan (1985) points out that an intermittent force with flexible spring action will occasionally produce semi-hyalinization on the pressure side and osteoclasts are formed below the hyalinized tissue so that bone resorption is less disturbed. In this way it is possible to produce a smooth and uniform movement if a small force is exerted and the appliance is worn regularly.

Functional appliances exert intermittent forces corresponding to the muscular movements that activate the appliance when short periods of pressure are applied to the teeth. Reitan (1985) states that '. . . it is not always possible to distinguish between the reactions evoked by loose and fixed removable appliances solely on the basis of the histologic findings'.

When it comes to the application of measurable forces to teeth in clinical treatment, Reitan (1985) advises that '. . . one can avoid formation of extensive hyalinization zones by applying a force below a 50 to 70 g threshold' and further, 'For movement of a small tooth it would be favourable to apply an initial force as light as 20 to 30 g'. These criteria are compatible with the rule suggested by Schwarz and, taken together, provide a practical baseline from which to move to the adjustment of pressure sources on removable appliances. It is also a simple matter to use a pressure gauge, in the mouth or on the bench, to measure the amount of pressure being exerted by any spring and so to be in a better position to interpret the clinical results produced by any appliance (*Figure 2.15*). The pull of

elastics can also be measured using the same instruments.

The patient's reaction to pressure on the teeth must be watched carefully. Patients vary in their reactions to pressure in the sense that some find that pressure, especially in the initial stages, produces discomfort and pain and complain accordingly. Excessive pressure can be immediately and intolerably painful. A pressure that is slightly too high, if maintained, can become very painful and the affected tooth sensitive to the lightest touch. Such a situation should not be allowed to develop as, apart from any warning signal that such pain might be, discomfort is a strong disincentive to cooperation in treatment. Orthodontic treatment should be carried out without discomfort to the patient and this can be achieved by proper adjustment of the appliance.

The effects of removable appliances

The effects produced by removable appliances are a result of the directions in which the forces developed by springs act on teeth and the ways in which teeth move under pressure.

The way in which a tooth moves under pressure depends on a number of factors such as whether the force applied to the tooth is aligned with the centre of resistance to movement, whether more than one force is being applied to the tooth, whether there is contact with an adjoining tooth, a baseplate or a stabilizing device. The stage of eruption also influences considerably the behaviour of a tooth when moved with a removable appliance.

It is commonly stated that removable appliances produce only 'simple tipping movements' of teeth with the possible implication that this is an undesirable limitation and it is likely that this criticism applies to mesiodistal movements where teeth incline together over an extraction site and may have a poor contact point relationship. This simplistic idea overlooks the fact that teeth are situated in the living tissues of the jaws and alveolar processes which, especially in the earlier years, grow and change as the teeth move or are moved. In a biological system like this there can be no such thing as a simple tipping movement. Movements produced by pressure on the crowns of teeth are reflected in the roots and, especially in the earlier years, teeth moved mesiodistally in this way usually show little tilting when treatment is completed and the occlusion has settled down. Furthermore, there are situations in which a tilting or inclining movement of a tooth is the correct movement needed in treatment (*Figures 2.16* and *2.17*).

The final effect is determined by the state of development of the occlusion, the amount of movement and the details of the masticatory relationship with its opponents of a tooth so moved.

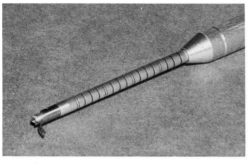

A

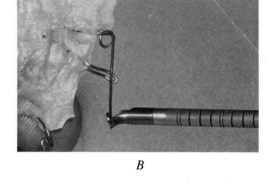

B

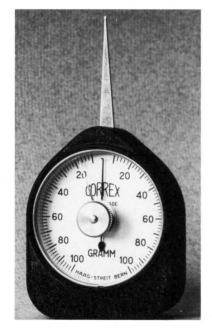

C

D

Figure 2.15 The use of pressure gauges; *A*, a plunger type of gauge calibrated in ounces. At the opposite end there is a hook which makes it possible to measure elastic tensions; *B*, measuring the pressure of a cantilever spring; *C*, the Correx pressure gauge calibrated in grammes; *D*, measuring the pressure of an apron spring

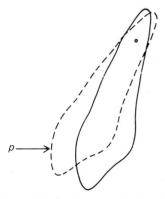

Figure 2.16 In a tooth which is tilted by means of an orthodontic pressure, tipping takes place about a point between the apex and the point at which pressure is applied

The springs used in removable appliances press on the smooth, hard enamel surfaces of the teeth and there is no friction or grip between the spring and the tooth. The effective pressure on a tooth can only be at right angles to the tooth surface at the point at which the spring is applied. If the spring acts in a direction which is not at right angles to the tooth surface, then the force exerted by the spring is resolved into two forces, one at right angles to the tooth surface which produces tooth movement and a second force parallel to the tooth surface which tends to depress the tooth. The reactions to these two resolved forces are absorbed respectively in the anchorage base and by the teeth to which the appliance is clasped (*Figure 2.18A*).

Springs should be applied to tooth surfaces accurately so that tooth movements take place in the directions that are intended. The direction in which

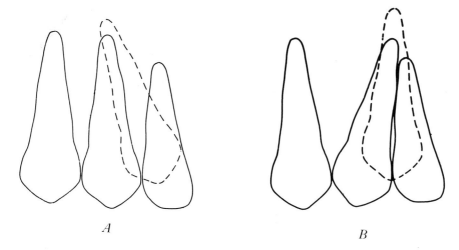

Figure 2.17 Favourable and unfavourable tipping of a tooth can be illustrated by the retroclination of an upper canine tooth; *A*, the canine apex is placed distally and the tooth, if tipped distally, lies favourably in the space available; *B*, the canine apex is mesially placed and moving the tooth into the space available increases an already unfavourable inclination. Broken line, before movement; continuous line, after movement

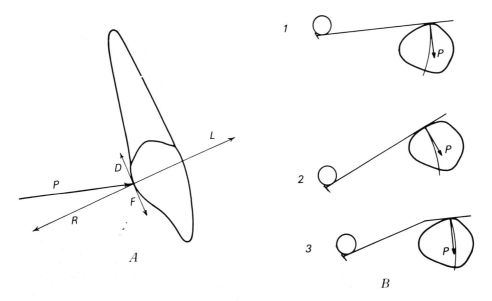

Figure 2.18 The action of springs on teeth; *A*, a spring exerting a pressure *P* on the lingual aspect of an upper incisor impinges on a sloping, frictionless surface. The effects of this force are to produce a force *L* at right angles to the surface impinged on, equal to the resolved part of the force *P* in this direction, tending to move the tooth labially; a force *F* parallel to the surface impinged on equal to the resolved part of the pressure *P* in this direction which tends to displace the appliance downwards. The reaction *R* to the force *L* tends also to displace the appliance in a downward and backward direction. In practice the appliance is the less movable element in the pressure system, being fixed to an anchorage, and the force *L* proclines the tooth and the reaction *D* to the force *F* tends to produce a depressing effect on the tooth; *B*, the point of fixation of a finger spring determines the direction in which it acts: *1*, the point of fixation is somewhat forward and the line of action is in a palatal direction; *2*, the point of fixation is somewhat backward and the line of action of the spring is in a buccal direction; *3*, the point of fixation is opposite the tooth and the spring is bent to make the point of applicatioin of pressure on the mesial surface, the line of action being distally in line with the buccal segment

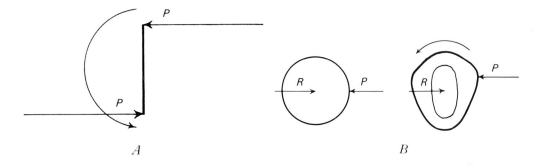

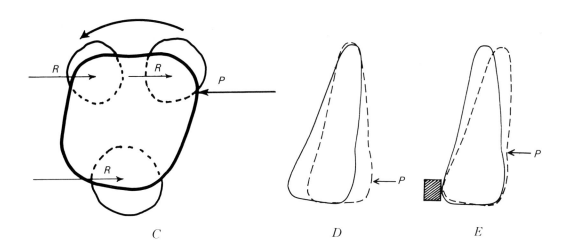

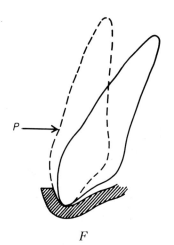

Figure 2.19 Rotation and root movement; *A*, the mechanical couple. Equal and opposite pressures which are not in line produce rotation; *B*, moment of a force about a point: *P* is the line of application of pressure, *R* is the centre of resistance. If the resistance is in line with the pressure, no rotation takes place. If the resistance is not in line with the pressure, rotation will occur. Pressing on the slightly buccally placed contact point of a premolar will produce rotation; *C*, in the case of an upper first molar, pressure on the mesial surface will produce rotation around the large palatal root; *D*, pressure *P* at the distal surface of an incisor that is free to move will produce mesial tipping; *E*, pressure *P* in a mesial direction at the distal gum margin of an incisor which is blocked at the mesial aspect of the incisal edge will produce mesial tipping of the root; *F*, pressure *P* at the labial gum margin of an incisor which is prevented from tipping at the incisal edge will produce root movement in a lingual direction

a spring is pressing on a tooth does not necessarily correspond with the arc in which the end of the spring is moving as the effective pressure on the tooth is at right angles to the tangent at the point on which the spring touches (*Figure 2.18B*).

It is important to align the force applied to a tooth with the centre of resistance to a movement if undesired rotation is to be avoided, but the rotational effect can be used to advantage when a tooth has rotated and moved forward following a tooth loss immediately mesially and this undesired movement has to be reversed. A simple pressure will produce the desired result.

Rotation and root movement

Rotation can be produced by the use of two equal and opposite forces which are offset to produce a mechanical couple. Upper central and lateral incisors can be rotated in this way (*Figure 2.19A*) (*see also Figure 5.5*). Premolar and molar teeth can also be rotated if pressure, offset from the centre of resistance to movement, is exerted on the tooth (*Figure 2.19B, C*).

A tooth must move as a whole or not at all but movement may be mainly at the crown or mainly at the apex or equally along the length of the tooth. Movement mainly at the apex is often referred to as 'root movement' and this effect can be produced by a removable appliance in certain circumstances.

If the crown of a tooth is prevented from moving mesiodistally or labiolingually by placing a fixed stabilizer such as a rigid wire or a baseplate so as to stabilize the crown, and pressure is applied to the tooth crown at or near the neck of the tooth, a mainly tilting movement of the root of the tooth will take place. Movement will not be as rapid as in moving the crown of the tooth, but mainly apical movement will be produced (*Figure 2.19D–F*) (*see also Figures 5.12, 5.13 and 5.14*).

Chapter 3

Labiolingual and buccolingual movement of teeth

The term 'labiolingual movement' applies to the anterior teeth, the incisors and canines, and buccolingual movement applies to the premolars and molars. In performing these movements an inclining effect is usually satisfactory and this can be performed by removable appliances in the great majority of cases.

Labial and buccal movement of teeth

Labial movement of incisors

This movement is called proclination of incisors while a similar movement of canine teeth and the teeth farther back is referred to as a labial and buccal movement.

Upper incisors may need to be proclined because of their biting lingually to the lower incisors; the fault may lie equally with the upper and with the lower teeth or may be mainly in the upper or in the lower teeth. It is important to assess and distinguish where the problem lies and to plan tooth movements so as to produce the necessary correction or improvement.

Lingual occlusion of upper incisors

The details of any case in point may vary considerably as shown in *Figures 3.1* and *3.2* illustrating two strongly contrasting instances. In the first case (*Figure 3.1*) there is a well-arranged dentition apart from the detail that one upper incisor is biting lingually to the lower incisors, overbite and overjet of the other anterior teeth being normal. In the second case (*Figure 3.2*) the lower labial segment, as a whole, occludes mesially to the upper and all the upper incisors bite lingually to the lower incisors. The differences between the two cases are of nature and degree. The second case contains problems of face size and shape that are not present in the first, and the discrepancy in the relationship of the incisor teeth is of a more severe degree in the second case than in the first. These are two extreme examples of upper incisors biting lingually to lower incisors and between them lie shades of discrepancy ranging from the mild to the extreme.

Factors which influence the correction of lingual occlusion of upper incisors to lower incisors are presented below.

Space conditions

If the upper anterior teeth are crowded, there may not be space to procline a lingually occluding upper tooth into line (*Figure 3.3A–D*).

Degree of overbite

If there is little overbite, upper incisors, when proclined, may not remain stable as overbite is further reduced by the movement of proclination (*Figure 3.4*).

Upper incisor inclination

If the upper incisors are already inclined forwards, proclination may further reduce overbite and leave the upper incisors in a traumatogenic position (*Figure 3.5*).

Dental base relationship

If there is a tendency to prenormality in the dental base relationship, there may be difficulty in achieving a correct incisor relationship by orthodontic means (*Figure 3.6*).

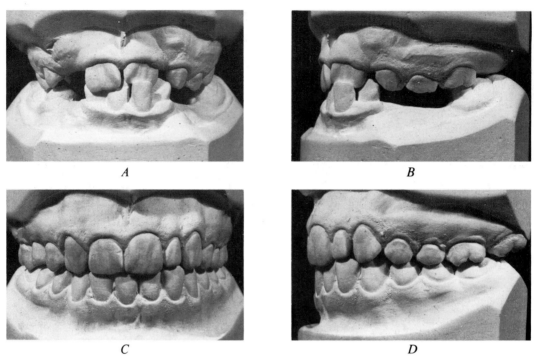

Figure 3.1. *A* and *B*, Front and side views of a patient aged 6 years with a single incisor caught behind the lower incisors; *C* and *D*, after proclination of the left upper central incisor, the dentition developed to an excellent arrangement apart from congenital absence of the right upper lateral incisor

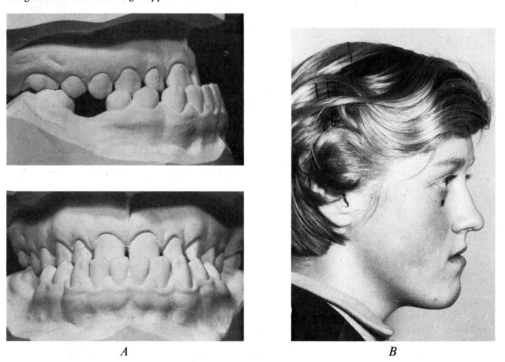

Figure 3.2. *A*, The upper incisors bite lingually to the lower incisors and so also do the canines; the underjet is 5 mm. This is a Class III malocclusion and in no way can incisor relation be corrected by purely orthodontic measures; *B*, this patient was treated by mandibular resection

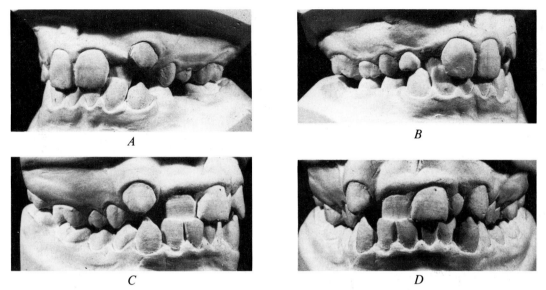

Figure 3.3 *A* and *B*, Right and left views of the patient with normal overbite and overjet of the upper central incisors. The upper lateral incisors bite lingually to the lower incisors, but there is not sufficient space to correct the lateral incisor positions; *C* and *D*, a similar case except that the upper right central and lateral incisors bite lingually to the lower incisors and there is insufficient space for correction of the lateral incisor

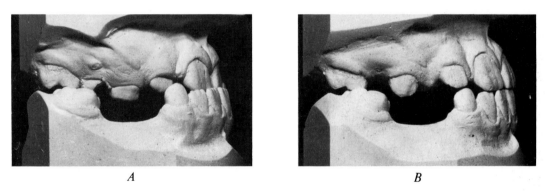

Figure 3.4 In this case the upper incisors have very little overbite (*A*) and after proclination (*B*) the overbite had disappeared completely and the upper incisors are in an unstable position. Retroclination of the lower incisors might help but would not be easy in the absence of space between the incisors or the extraction of the lower premolars which are not as yet erupted

Mandibular displacement

Where an upper incisor or a number of upper incisors bite lingually to the lower incisors, the possibility of there being a forward deviation, displacement or posturing of the mandible on closing from the rest position to occlusion should be looked for. If there is such a displacement forwards and the patient can bring the lower incisors edge-to-edge with the upper incisor or incisors, treatment of the case may be simplified as part of the correction will be produced by the mandible's

closing to occlusion without shifting forwards from the abnormal or premature contact of the incisor teeth (*Figure 3.7*).

Dental base discrepancy and inadequate overbite relationship produce the greatest problems in the stability of corrected incisor relationship. The following case histories illustrate some of the problems encountered in correcting upper incisors which bite lingually to the lower incisors.

Figure 3.8 shows a developing normal dentition apart from the lingual occlusion of a single incisor. Arch form was excellent, space conditions were

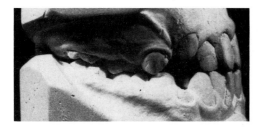

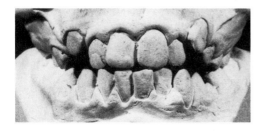

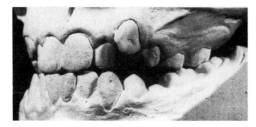

Figure 3.5 This patient has not only crowding but also no overbite so that correction of the upper lateral incisors requires space. It can be seen that the lower incisors appear retroclined so that there is not a good prospect for producing a good overbite relationship. This patient would probably, in due course, require surgical treatment

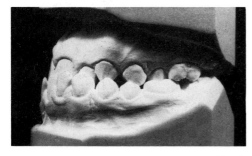

Figure 3.6 This patient has some degree of overbite, but the dental base discrepancy suggests that the stability of the upper incisors after correction might be in doubt. Note that the buccal segment relationship is markedly prenormal

adequate, overbite and overjet normal. Treatment was to procline the affected tooth with an appliance using a single finger spring of 0.5 mm thickness, guarded to hold the spring down against the tooth. The presence of a space betweeen the central incisors made possible the placing of the guard in a vertical position and projecting adequately to cover the full range of action of the spring. Even though there was little overbite, bite-planes were placed over the posterior teeth while the incisor tooth was being moved.

Figures 3.9 and *3.10* show two cases of single central incisor teeth caught behind the bite in patients of 10 and 13 years of age. The dentitions were otherwise normal and there were no problems of space, overbite relationship or dental base discrepancy. Single cantilever springs were used in each case (*Figure 3.11*), the bite being propped temporarily on bite-planes covering the back teeth. There was no problem of stability of the treated result. It is interesting to observe the faceting on the lingually placed upper incisors. The wear can be seen on careful examination of the photographs.

In *Figure 3.12* are seen the casts of a young patient with crowding of the incisors, the lateral incisors being caught behind the bite of the lower incisors. In this case, the deciduous canine tooth on the patient's right side was removed before correcting the lateral incisors because of the lack of space.

The older patient should not despair of treatment of misplaced incisor teeth. The patient illustrated in *Figure 3.13* was 45 years of age and was referred for advice prior to the construction of prostheses to replace posterior teeth. The misplaced upper central incisors were moved without difficulty into stable positions by means of a double cantilever spring in conjunction with bite-planes on the teeth in the buccal segments. Similar appliances for performing such a movement are shown in *Figure 3.14*.

In the case shown in *Figure 3.15* it was necessary to procline four upper incisors into correct relationship with the lower incisors. Here again, the space conditions were adequate and overjet and overbite were normal. As the teeth were not spaced, it was not possible to carry the guide for the spring forwards beyond the teeth. If the spring shows a tendency to slip down and under the incisors, the spring may be activated a little upwards as well as forwards as this counteracts any tendency for the spring to slip out of contact with the teeth. *Figure 3.16* shows a similar case.

Figure 3.17 shows a young patient with normal buccal occlusion but minimal overbite. When the upper left central and lateral incisors were proclined, they matched the right central and lateral incisors which were already in normal occlusion, although having little or no overbite relation with the lower incisors. The patient shown in *Figure 3.18* was older, being 26 years of age, and when the

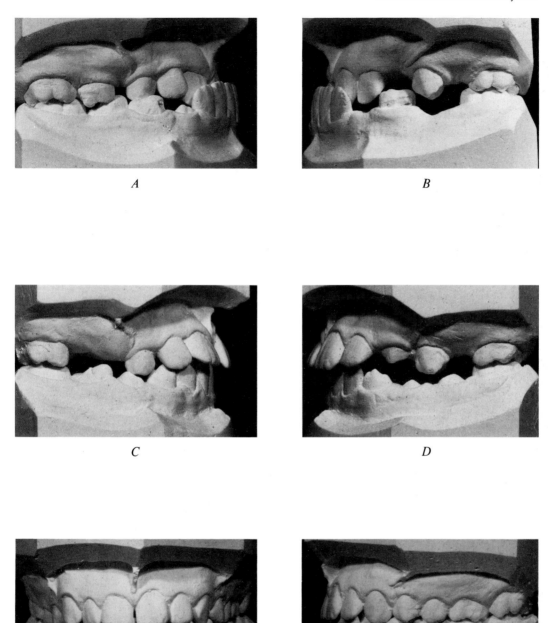

Figure 3.7 This patient has, apparently, a fairly severe dental base discrepancy but note that at *A* and *B* the molar relationship is normal. After correction of the incisor relationship by proclination of the upper incisors (*C* and *D*) note the change in the molar relation indicating that there has been a postural element in the incisor discrepancy. At *E* and *F* the occlusion has developed normally and there has been improvement in the upper incisor inclination

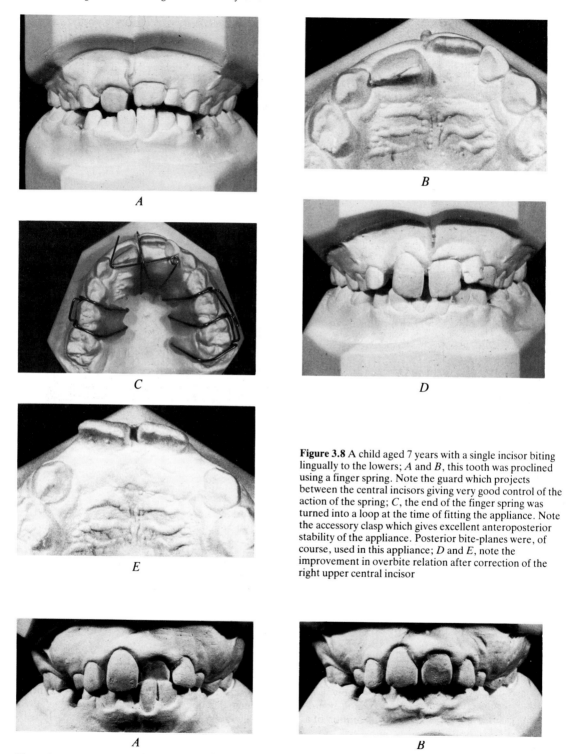

A

B

C

D

E

Figure 3.8 A child aged 7 years with a single incisor biting lingually to the lowers; *A* and *B*, this tooth was proclined using a finger spring. Note the guard which projects between the central incisors giving very good control of the action of the spring; *C*, the end of the finger spring was turned into a loop at the time of fitting the appliance. Note the accessory clasp which gives excellent anteroposterior stability of the appliance. Posterior bite-planes were, of course, used in this appliance; *D* and *E*, note the improvement in overbite relation after correction of the right upper central incisor

A

B

Figure 3.9 *A*, An excellent occlusion with one incisor behind the bite in a patient aged 9 years; *B*, the incisor was corrected by means of a finger spring on an appliance clasped as shown with posterior bite-planes. The presence of a space between the incisors permitted the use of a guard which came forwards between the teeth giving excellent control of the spring's action

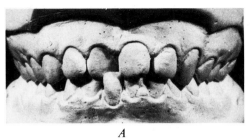

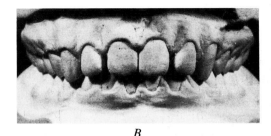

A   *B*

Figure 3.10 *A*, Another, somewhat older, patient having the right upper central incisor caught lingually to the right lower central incisor. The bite was propped on the posterior teeth and the offending incisor proclined sufficiently to correct the malocclusion

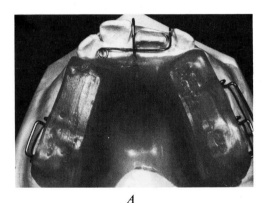

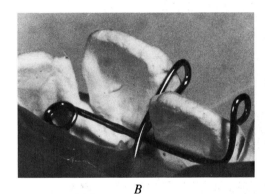

A   *B*

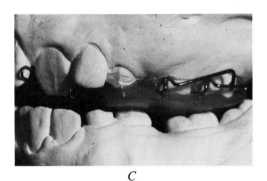

Figure 3.11 The appliance which was used in treating the patient in *Figure 3.10*; *A*, the layout of the spring, clasps and biting planes. Note that the guard passes forwards between the central incisors thereby controlling the action of the spring; *B*, close-up of the spring. Note the looped end of the spring and how it does not interfere with the adjoining tooth; *C*, the bite-planes are curved to fit the line of the upper occlusal plane. Note the accessory arrowhead for anteroposterior stability

C

upper central incisors were proclined into correct occlusion, the overbite was reduced but adequate to maintain correct incisor relationship.

The last two cases in this category show how surprising results are achieved in apparently unpromising cases. *Figure 3.19* shows the dentition of a child of 8 years of age just as the upper incisors are beginning to erupt. First, the centrals were proclined into correct relationship to the lower incisors and the lateral incisors had also to be corrected shortly after their eruption. The dentition then proceeded to develop normally. *Figure 3.20* shows a

girl of 7 years of age in whom a very unpromising incisor relationship improved spontaneously, and as the lower incisors were slightly spaced, correction of the incisor relationship was effected by slightly proclining the upper incisors and retroclining the lower incisors. The dentition thereafter developed normally.

Labial movement of lower incisors

Proclination of lower incisors is a movement which today is undertaken very much less often than

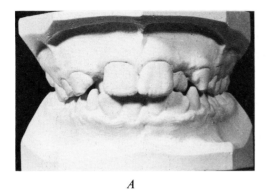

A

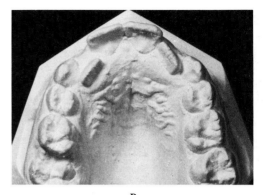

B

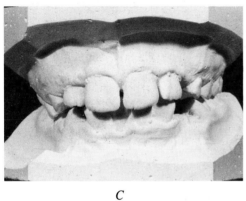

C

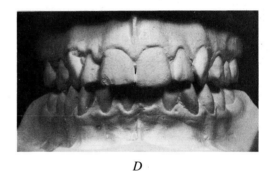

D

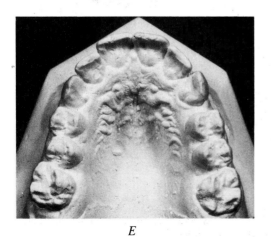

E

Figure 3.12 *A* and *B*, A young patient aged 8 years in whom the upper lateral incisors were biting lingually to the lower incisors. This patient had an underlying crowding problem and there was not room to procline the upper lateral incisors; *C*, treatment necessitated removal of the upper deciduous canines followed by proclination of the lateral incisors. The crowding problem was treated by removal of first permanent molars which had very large fillings; *D* and *E*, result at 14 years of age

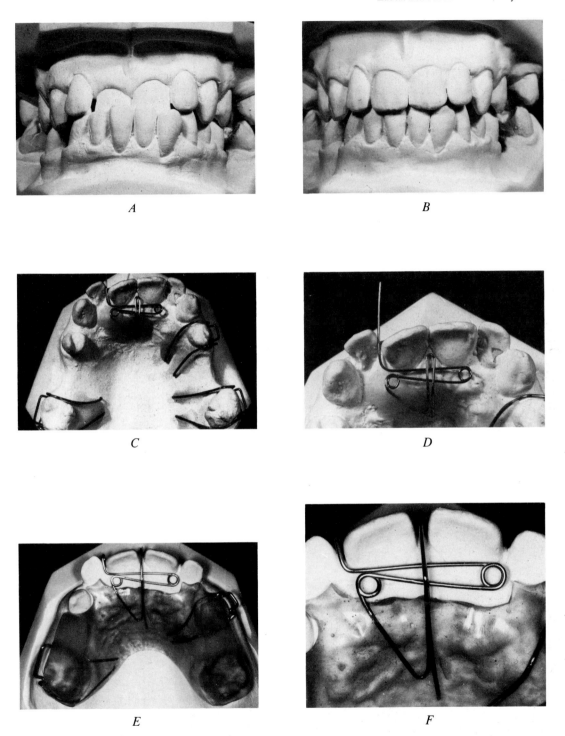

Figure 3.13 *A*, This is an older patient aged about 45 years who, surprisingly, did not have the upper central incisors corrected in childhood. Before the construction of prostheses, the upper central incisors were corrected with a double cantilever spring, *C* and *D*. The end of the spring was turned into a loop at the time of fitting the appliance. Posterior bite-planes were used; *B*, shows the completed orthodontic result. Where the incisors are spaced, the guard controlling the spring can be brought between the teeth so obtaining better control of the spring, *E* and *F*

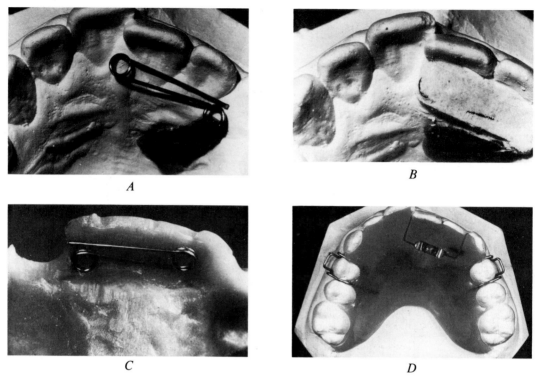

Figure 3.14 Some alternative ways of proclining upper incisors; *A*, a double cantilever spring which is boxed in; *B*, the spring is encased in plaster and a flat surface formed on top of the plaster. The baseplate is then brought over the spring as shown in *C*. *D*, a screw is sometimes convenient as it can be activated by the patient

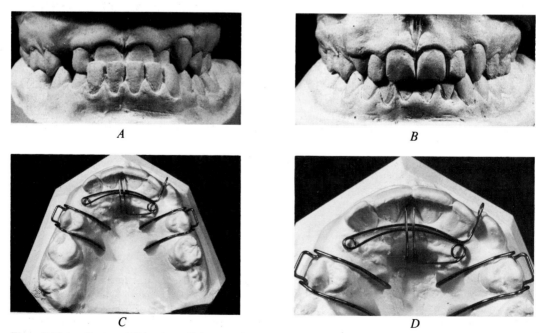

Figure 3.15 A patient aged 12 in whom all the upper incisors occluded lingually to the lower incisors. The bite was propped on posterior bite-planes and a double cantilever spring (*C* and *D*) was used to procline all four teeth simultaneously; *A*, before treatment, *B*, after treatment

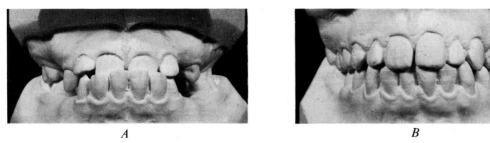

Figure 3.16 *A*, A similar case to the previous one involving three incisors; *B*, in this case, the right upper canine had to be removed but the right upper first premolar resembles the canine sufficiently

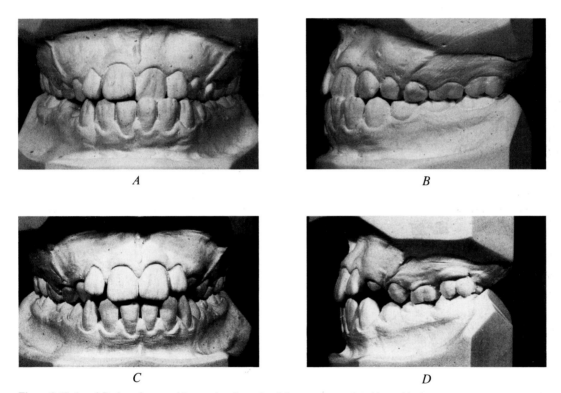

Figure 3.17 *A* and *B*, A patient aged 8 years in whom the right upper central and lateral incisors occluded normally with an absolute minimum of overbite and the left upper central and lateral incisors bite lingually to the lower incisors; *C* and *D*, these teeth were proclined slightly to match the upper right incisors exactly. It is possible that the overbite has improved very slightly but the ultimate stability of the anterior labial segment will remain to be seen

formerly. Indeed, such are often felt to be the later disadvantages of proclining lower incisors that it might be concluded that this movement is totally undesirable. There may, however, occasionally be circumstances in which this movement is required and it is possible to produce it using a removable appliance. The recommended removable appliance resembles the fixed lower lingual arch with apron springs which was formerly used to produce this tooth movement. The removable appliance consists of a lingual arch with apron springs attached by welding a tape loop or held by an attachment embedded in the baseplate (*Figure 3.21*).

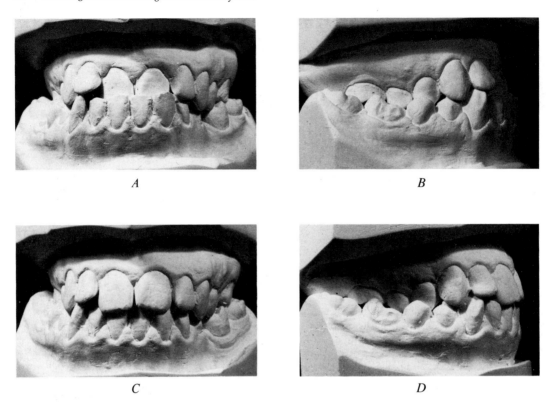

A   *B*

C   *D*

Figure 3.18 *A* and *B*, An older patient in whom the upper central incisors bite lingually to the lower incisors and when corrected the overbite on the teeth which had been moved was markedly reduced; *C* and *D*, it does seem, however, that the overbite will be sufficient to maintain stability of the corrected incisor relationship

Labial movement of upper canine teeth

The treatment of the palatally inclined upper canine tooth can be satisfactory if the position of the apex of the tooth is normal and the tooth only requires to be inclined in a labial direction. Misplacement of the permanent upper canine tooth is a complex subject and it is only possible here to outline the nature of the problems connected with management of such cases. Accurate assessment of the ectopic upper canine is important as a number of factors can create difficulties in treatment.

Misplacement of the canine apex

The apex of the canine may be displaced from its proper position as well as the crown. This will create difficulties in bringing the tooth into good alignment.

Space conditions in the dental arch

There may be delay in eruption of the permanent canine and in bringing it into alignment. In the meantime, the deciduous canine is smaller than the permanent canine and cannot maintain the amount of space needed for a permanent tooth.

Rotation of the permanent canine

Displaced canines may be rotated more or less severely, adding an extra dimension to the treatment procedure.

Failure of eruption

A buried canine which does not erupt at the proper time may fail in the end to erupt fully to the occlusal level of the other teeth. The longer treatment is delayed, the greater the possibility that the canine will lose its capacity for eruption.

The lingually placed canine, after exposure, may be moved in a labial direction using a clasped removable appliance. It is necessary to envisage the path which the canine crown is to move along and to arrange the point of fixation of the spring and the

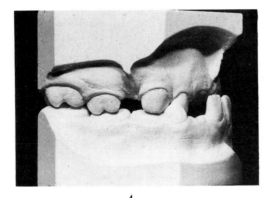

A

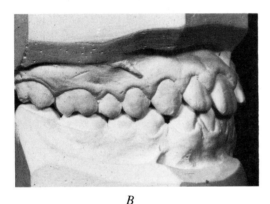

B

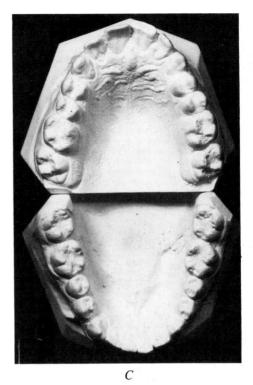

C

Figure 3.19 *A*, A boy aged 8 years in whom the upper central incisors are just beginning to erupt. The incisor relation seems most unpromising but these teeth and subsequently the lateral incisors were proclined leading to the development of normal occlusion at 12 years of age. The left upper central was fractured in a bicycle accident; *B* and *C*, lateral and occlusal views at 14 years of age

point of application of pressure with great care. If the canine crown is much displaced, it may not be necessary to prop the bite until the tooth has actually been moved and comes into contact with the lower teeth. When this point arrives, the bite should be propped to allow the canine tooth to move easily across the bite of the lower teeth. As already mentioned, such teeth are frequently rotated and the rotation of the tooth into correct alignment (a procedure sometimes referred to as 'derotation') can be done by means of a fixed/removable appliance combination using an attachment bonded to the canine tooth.

One of the important aspects of the treatability of such cases is the vertical position of the tooth in relation to the adjoining teeth. The position of the crown of the tooth may be short of the occlusal plane owing to the tooth having formed completely before being moved into position and therefore not, in the end, erupting fully. Orthodontic elongation of such a tooth is a procedure to be undertaken with circumspection (*Figures 3.22, 3.23* and *3.24*).

Labial movement of lower canines

This movement is not often needed as a single tooth movement but if necessary can be done with an apron spring attached to a lingual arch or by means of a finger spring.

Buccal movements of upper and lower premolars and molars

These movements can be done quite effectively using clasped removable appliances by means of finger springs and double cantilever springs. Because of the close proximity of the tongue to the buccal teeth, springs in this region must be very neatly made with small coils so that the tongue does not bulge into the area of the spring and become caught. Such springs are sometimes boxed in by the baseplate to avoid this possible source of trouble, but in turn this creates difficulties which outweigh any possible advantages; that is to say the cavities

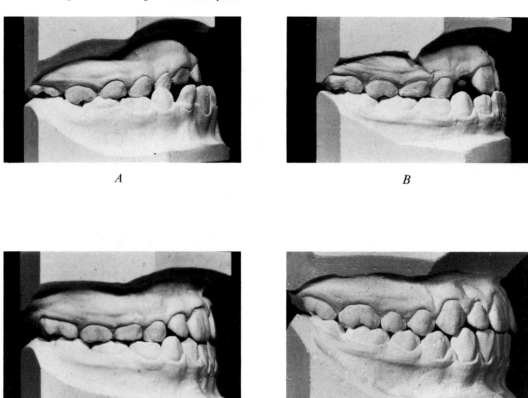

A   *B*

C   *D*

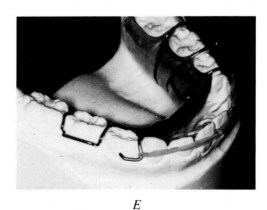

E

Figure 3.20 *A*, A girl aged 7 years in whom the occlusal relation tended markedly to prenormality; *B*, after a period of observation, the incisor relation had improved considerably and at this stage the upper incisors were proclined a little and the lower incisors retroclined using an elastic stretched between hooks and the incisor relation became corrected (*C*); *D*, the occlusion developed to normal with a slight prenormal tendency; *E* shows the lower appliance;

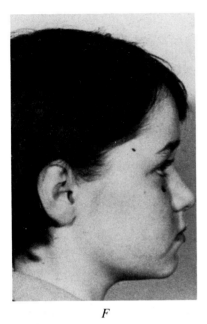

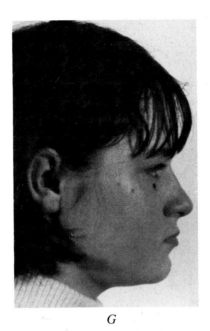

F   G

Figure 3.20 continued *F* and *G* show the appearance of the profile at 8 and at 18 years of age

beneath the plate act as food traps and the covering up of the spring renders its manipulation and adjustment unduly difficult. The more open the spring can be, the more easy it is to keep clean and to adjust (*Figure 3.25A* and *B*).

In the lower arch, a cantilever spring of 0.6 mm wire wound on a support is very effective for buccal movement of single teeth (*Figure 3.25C* and *D*).

There is one useful spring which it is necessary to cover up in the way described with the disadvantages being accepted. This is a spring known as a 'T' spring or 'club' spring which is efficient in buccal movement of upper molars and premolars (*Figure 3.25E*). This spring is covered by the baseplate but its adjustment is done by lifting the spring away from the baseplate. Cleanliness must be carefully attended to.

The buccolingual movement of molars and premolars must be undertaken with due regard to their ultimate stability, and here the width dimensions of the upper and lower arches and the sharpness and interdigitations of the cusps of the teeth are factors which influence the treatability of the condition (*Figures 3.26, 3.27* and *3.28*).

Buccolingual adjustment of one or two teeth will involve consideration of the alignment of the buccal segments as a whole, from which it may appear that one or two teeth are, in fact, displaced buccally or lingually and are, therefore, amenable to permanent correction in the alignment of the arch. The question of the buccolingual movement of entire dental arches is properly considered under the heading of arch expansion which will be dealt with in Chapter 6.

It frequently happens that when a tooth in the buccal segments needs to be corrected buccolingually, an opposing tooth also needs to be moved as part of the correction (*see below* Lingual movement of molars and premolars).

Lingual movement of teeth

Upper incisors

Retroclination of upper incisors is frequently called for and can be carried out in a number of ways. It is important to consider the relationship of these teeth to the lower incisors and also to the adjoining tissues of the lips and tongue as well as considering the dental base relationship.

In a straightforward case, the dental base relationship and soft tissue morphology are normal and retroclination of the upper incisors will produce a normal relationship of the crowns of the upper and lower incisors. The soft tissues of the lips and tongue will then adapt themselves in such a way as to maintain the stability of the relationship of the incisor teeth at the end of treatment.

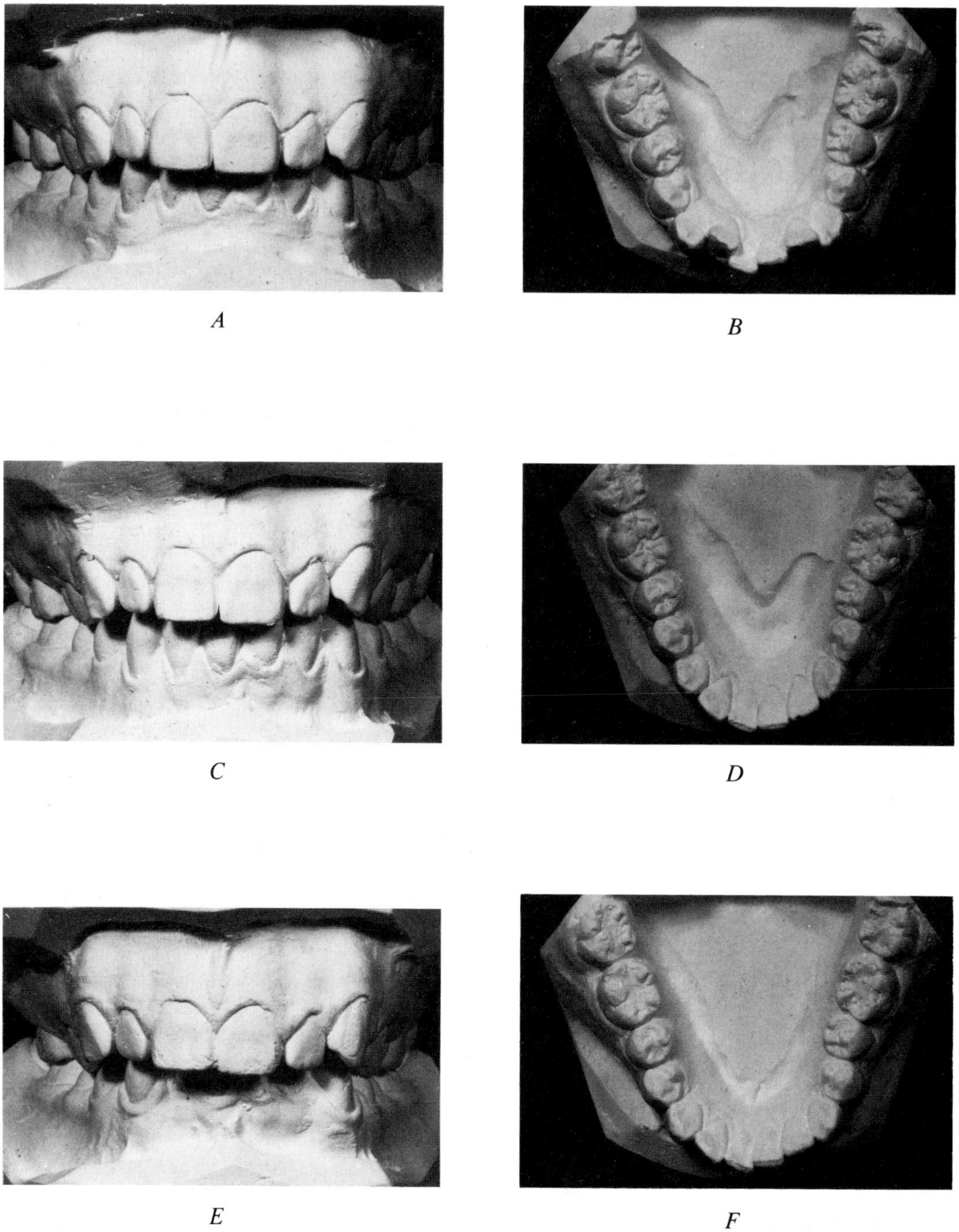

A

B

C

D

E

F

Figure 3.21 *A* and *B*, This patient, aged 12 years, had an excellent upper arch and crowding in the lower labial segment; *C* and *D*, the bite was opened using a Sved bite-plane and the lower incisors aligned using apron springs on a lower removable lingual arch; *E* and *F*, the new incisor relationship settled well and lower third molars were removed. Upper third molars were congenitally absent;

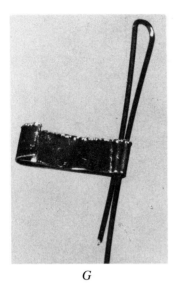

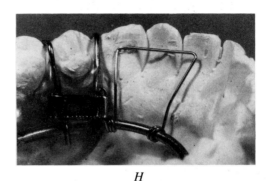

G   H

Figure 3.21 continued *G* and *H*, the lower appliance. The spring wire was held with a tape loop embedded in the baseplate

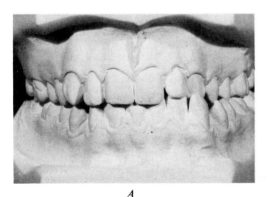

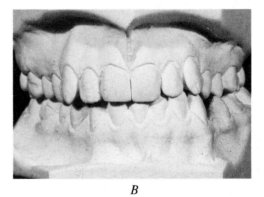

A   B

Figure 3.22 Correction of the left permanent canines by lingual movement of the lower and labial movement of the upper. The patient has a lower midline shift to the left and overbite of the treated canine teeth is minimal but the condition proved stable and considerably enhanced the patient's appearance; *A*, before treatment; *B*, after treatment

One of the traditional methods for applying pressure on the labial surfaces of the upper incisors is by means of apron springs wound on a high labial archwire made of heavy gauge wire which is attached to a baseplate. The archwire is an extension of the baseplate and contributes little to the flexibility of the system. The apron springs are of fine gauge wire, 0.3 mm thick, having three or four coils which give a very flexible spring but, at the same time, a spring which resists interferences from the lips and from food during eating. The baseplate is clasped usually to the first molar teeth and can have, if necessary, auxiliary clasps on the second premolars (*Figure 3.29*). Apron springs of this kind have the great advantage that they can be adjusted to produce different effects on the individual teeth but, if required, such an apron spring can be made wide enough to act on two teeth. By placing a coil

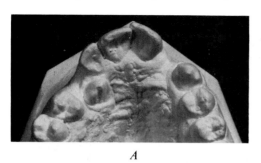

A

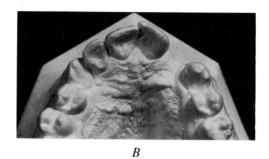

B

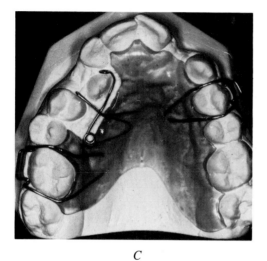

C

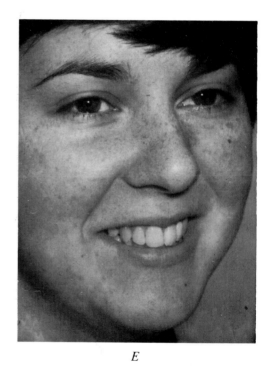

E

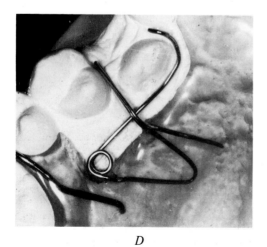

D

Figure 3.23 Correction of unerupted and palatally displaced right upper canine in a patient aged 14 years. This tooth was unerupted but was exposed surgically and came to the position shown in *A*. The tooth was moved to the position shown in *B* with the appliance seen in *C* and *D*. Of necessity the left upper lateral incisor was removed because of pulp death with invagination at the cingulum; *E*, the treatment was completed by constructing a bridge for the extracted lateral incisor

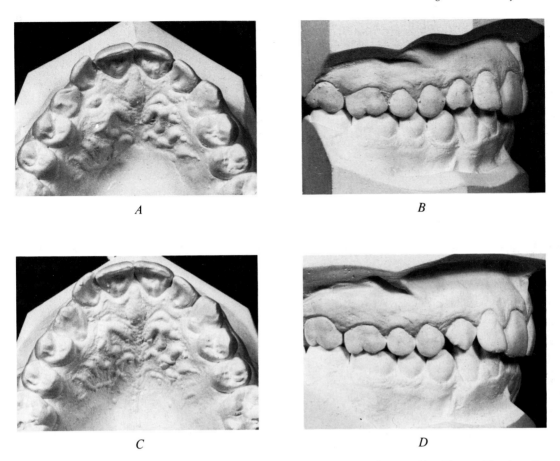

A   B

C   D

Figure 3.24 *A* and *B*, correction of the right upper canine tooth which had recently erupted in a 25-year-old patient. *C* and *D*, the canine was moved into line following extraction of the right upper deciduous canine, replacing the deciduous with a permanent tooth

system at each end of an apron spring of this kind, the spring can be made wide enough to act on three or four teeth.

The Roberts retraction appliance for the upper anterior teeth (Roberts, 1956; *Figure 3.30*) is unobtrusive and effective. The appliance acts on the whole labial segment and effects on individual teeth are not easy to obtain.

Neither the high labial bow and apron spring nor the Roberts retractor is entirely convenient for the retroclination of a single incisor or to apply pressure to a single incisor as, for instance, when producing rotation. A much simpler arrangement is to use a self-supporting spring which is brought from a distal point, a little farther back on the arch, and is formed into a loop at the active end which lies against the tooth which is to be retroclined. Such a spring is unobtrusive and easy to wear and adjust and produces a very satisfactory movement of the tooth in a lingual direction (*Figure 3.31*).

In most cases, but not all, it is necessary first to retract canine teeth after creation of space by extraction farther back in the arch (*see* Mesiodistal movement of teeth, p. 49).

Figures 3.32–3.36 illustrate various aspects of lingual movement of upper incisors.

Lingual movement of canines

Upper and lower canines, which are prominent and which lie opposite an existing space in the arch or a space which has been created by extraction, can be moved lingually into such a space by means of a spring made like a self-supporting canine retractor with the acting end lying on the labial surface of the tooth. The spring is activated in a lingual direction. A self-supporting canine retractor can be adjusted to act in this way by turning the end through 90°.

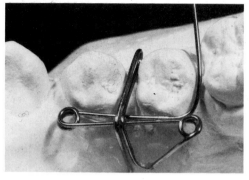

A

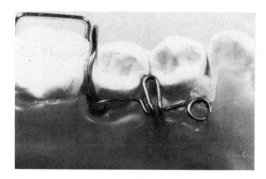

B

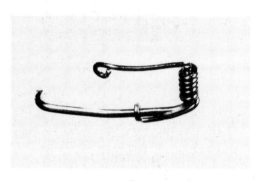

C

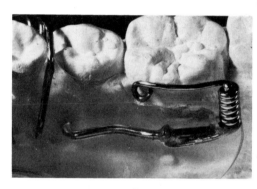

D

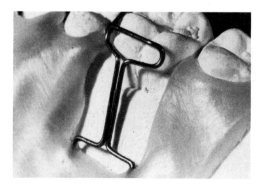

E

Figure 3.25 Buccal movement of premolars and molars; *A*, double cantilever spring to move left upper first and second molar labially. Note that there is space between the teeth to carry the guard well outwards to control the spring. When fitting the appliance, the end of the spring is turned into a loop; *B*, a single cantilever spring to move left lower second premolar buccally. Note that the spring is cranked as it was not possible to carry the guard between the teeth and cranking the spring keeps it better under the guard; *C* and *D*, a supported spring to move a lower molar buccally. The spring is of 0.6 mm wire wound on a support 1.0 mm thick. The spring is soldered or welded to the support and then wound. Note the rounded end of the spring; *E*, a torque spring to move an upper molar buccally. The transverse sections act as torque springs giving the spring considerable flexibility. This spring is boxed in order to make the baseplate adequately strong but is shown here before plastering and boxing

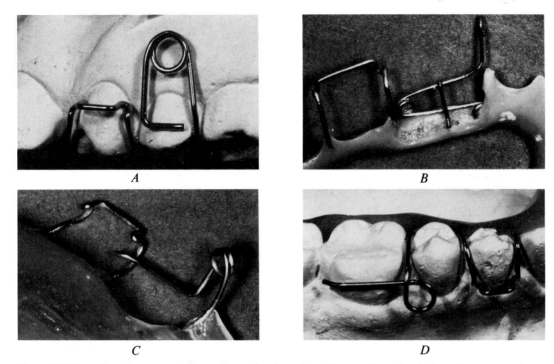

Figure 3.26 Buccolingual movement of premolars and molars; *A*, a self-supporting spring for lingual movement of premolar; *B*, double cantilever spring for buccal movement of two premolars; *C*, self-supporting spring for lingual movement of two premolars; *D*, self-supporting spring for lingual movement of molar

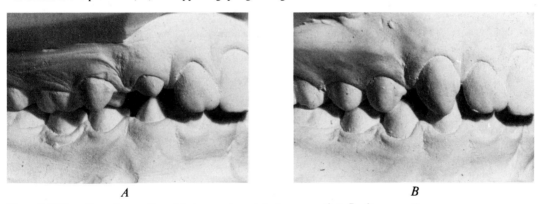

Figure 3.27 Buccolingual correction of first premolars; *A*, before correction; *B*, after correction

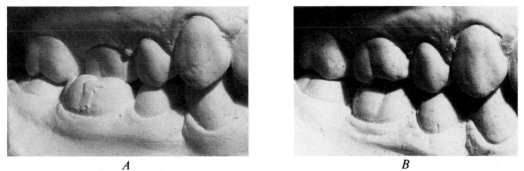

Figure 3.28 Buccolingual correction of first molars; *A*, before correction; *B*, after correction

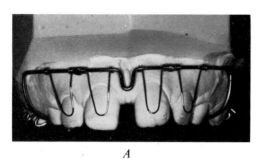

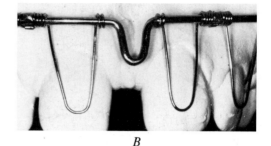

Figure 3.29 *A*, Appliance for lingual movement of upper incisors with 1.0 mm archwire and apron springs; *B*, the springs are attached by tape to the archwire (*see* Welding). It is also possible to attach the springs by soldering

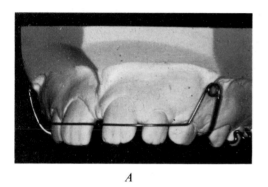

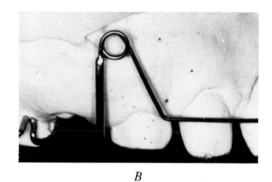

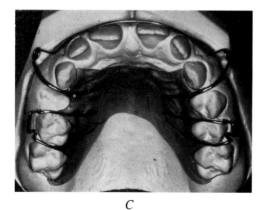

Figure 3.30 The Roberts retractor. *A* and *B*, the apron spring is made of 0.5 mm wire supported in tubes of softened stainless steel; *C*, anchorage is gained from the teeth in the buccal segments and the baseplate is cut away to allow the incisors to retrocline

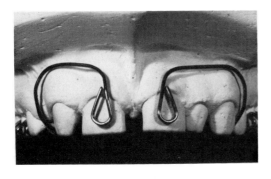

Figure 3.31 Single self-supporting springs for lingual movement of upper incisors. The springs are of 0.7 mm wire and the ends are formed into loops which are smooth to the inner surface of the cheeks and lips

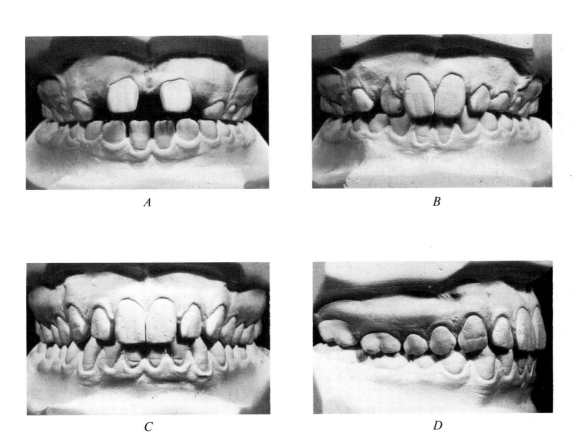

A

B

C

D

Figure 3.32 A patient aged 8 years who sucked her thumb and had a grade 2 fraenum labii; *A*, before treatment; *B*, a fraenectomy was done and an appliance with self-supporting springs was used to retrocline the upper central incisors. The appliance also acted as a substitute for the thumb. Thumb sucking was thereafter discontinued; *C* and *D*, the occlusion developed normally and the patient had excellent arch form and normal occlusion

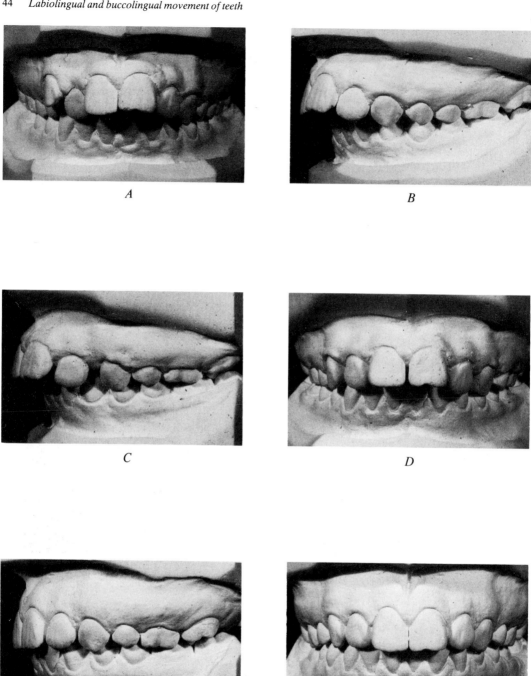

Figure 3.33 A patient aged 12 years who had a Class II division 1 malocclusion. This was treated by extraction of the upper first premolars, retraction of the canines and lingual inclination of the incisor teeth; *A* and *B*, before treatment; *C* and *D*, first premolars extracted, canines moved distally; *E* and *F*, treatment complete

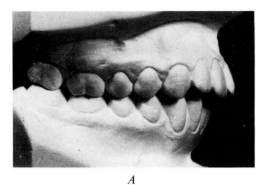

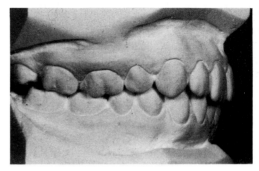

A   B

Figure 3.34. A patient aged 20 years who had a Class II division 1 malocclusion. This was treated by extraction of first premolars and retraction of canines and incisor teeth; *A*, before; *B*, after

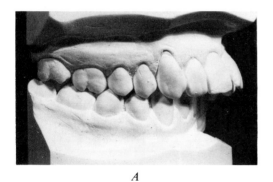

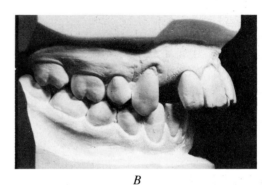

A   B

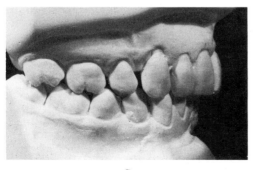

C

Figure 3.35 *A*, A young adult female with severe Class II division 1 malocclusion. The overbite was complete and was reduced by means of a Sved plate after which the first premolars were extracted; *B*, the canines have been retracted; *C*, the labial segment has now been retroclined. The condition remained stable and, as a final stage of treatment, the canine teeth were rotated mesiolingually as they were showing the mesial surfaces and had a pointed appearance. The patient maintained a very high standard of oral hygiene and was producing erosion of the gum margins at the canine teeth but was warned about appropriate oral care

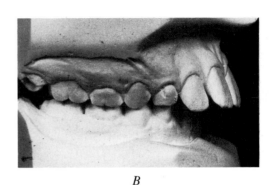

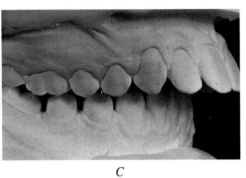

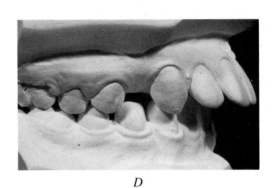

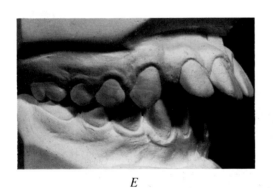

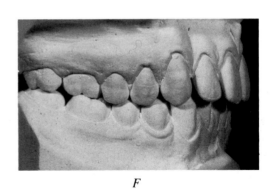

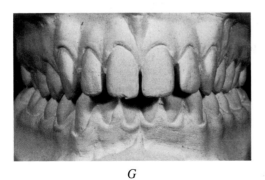

A

B

C

D

E

F

G

Figure 3.36 *A* and *B*, A young boy with a very pronounced
Class II division 1 malocclusion. The first premolars had
very heavy fillings. The lower first molars were extracted at
the age of 10 years and the spaces closed very rapidly, *C*.
At age 12 years the overbite was reduced by means of a
Sved plate and the upper first permanent molars were
removed and the premolars retracted into normal
relationship with the lower premolars, *D*; the canines were
then retracted *E–H*; and the upper anterior teeth
retroclined, *I–K* portraits at age 8 and age 18

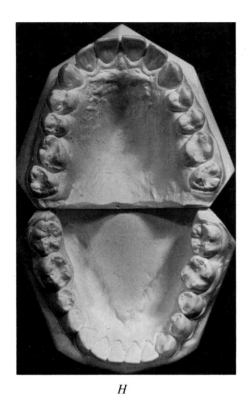

H

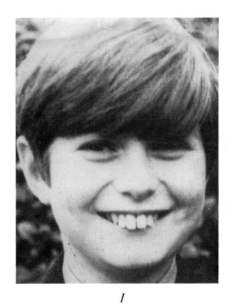

I

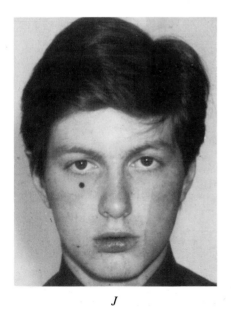

J

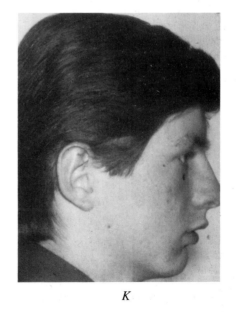

K

Figure 3.36 continued

Lingual movement of molars and premolars

There is little space in the buccal segments for the placement of arches for the support of springs so that in this area lingual movement must be carried out by means of self-supporting springs.

Such springs need to be attached to the baseplate and brought across the occlusal surfaces of the embrasures so that great care must be taken that the tag of the spring does not impede the lingual movement of the tooth and, naturally enough, the baseplate must be cut away sufficiently to allow the tooth to move. There is not too great a problem in the upper arch where the baseplate runs down to the middle line, but in the lower arch the baseplate must be left adequately thick for easing away from the tooth and the easing must be carried right down well beyond the gum margin. The active end of the spring begins with a coil for additional flexibility and the arm of the spring is laid against the buccal side of the tooth and activated in a lingual direction. It is possible in this way to move one molar or two premolars with a single spring.

Springs for lingual movement of premolars may also be constructed like the self-supporting canine retractor and can also be made to move two premolars (*see Figure 3.26*).

Chapter 4

Mesiodistal movement of teeth

Labio- and buccolingual tiltings of teeth do not usually produce untoward effects; the inclinations which result are, as a rule, corrections of misalignments. The mesiodistal alignment of the teeth is important to the interproximal contact relationships of the teeth and mesiodistal tiltings, whether occurring naturally or as a result of orthodontic tooth movement, can lead to poor approximal contacts, unfavourable functional alignment of tooth axes and, in the anterior region, an undesirable appearance of the teeth.

Mesiodistal inclination of the teeth can, therefore, be seen from the point of view of wrong inclinations that can be simply corrected by tilting teeth into correct alignment by a removable appliance, or as a mesiodistal movement which may produce an undesirable inclination of the tooth being moved.

The need for making mesiodistal movements arises in the alignment of the dental arch, there being space either occurring naturally or created by extraction of a tooth or of teeth. Such movement may be required at any point in the dental arch from the incisor region to the neighbourhood of the second and third molar teeth.

The most effective way of moving teeth mesiodistally is by the use of a palatal finger spring suitably guarded and guided and placed so that the line of action of the spring is along the line of the dental arch. This entails some care in placing the point of attachment of the spring and this detail is too often neglected in the construction of appliances.

Mesiodistal movement of incisors

In the incisor region, the need for mesiodistal movement often occurs when there is spacing due to the absence of teeth, such as the lateral incisors, or due to damage to a tooth, usually a central incisor, leading to its loss. The adjustment of the space available to make possible the placing of an artificial tooth is the usual requirement and when front teeth are moved mesiodistally by means of a removable appliance this always produces tilting of the tooth (*Figures 4.1* and *4.2*). If the tilting corrects an otherwise undesirable inclination, this is all to the good (*Figure 4.3*), but often the movement of the crown into a position to make possible the placing of an artificial tooth tilts the tooth that is moved, producing an unpleasant appearance due to the inclination of the incisal edge and possibly an abnormal contact with the adjoining tooth (*Figure 4.4*).

The ideal answer to this problem is to use a multiband appliance to rearrange the teeth as this gives control also of the axial inclinations. It is, however, possible to correct axial inclinations of anterior teeth with removable appliances if they are not rotated (*see* Rotation and root movement of teeth, Chapter 5).

Mesiodistal movement of canines

The distal movement of upper canine teeth can usually be done by palatal finger springs (*Figure 4.5A*), but sometimes needs to be done by a buccally placed, self-supporting spring of 0.7 mm wire. This spring is useful at any time but is particularly so when the canine overlaps the lateral incisor and is not easily accessible from the lingual side of the arch (*Figure 4.5B* and *C*).

The plain or standard buccal canine retractor is perfectly satisfactory if adjusted with care, but can be further improved by the addition of a stabilizer

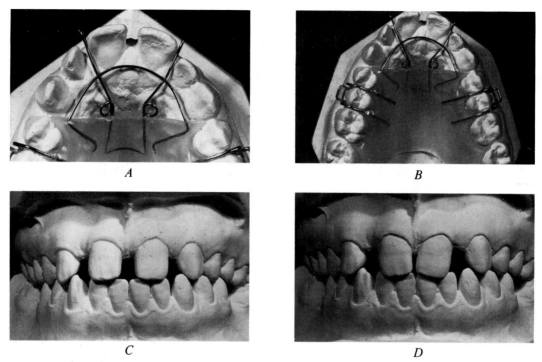

Figure 4.1 *A* and *B*, Palatal finger springs to approximate the upper central incisors. Note the point of attachment of the springs and the manner in which they are brought round to the distal surfaces of the teeth. Pressures used are equal and opposite so giving reciprocal anchorage; *C* and *D*, the teeth are moved together but incline slightly. The apices of the teeth are moved together as shown in Chapter 5

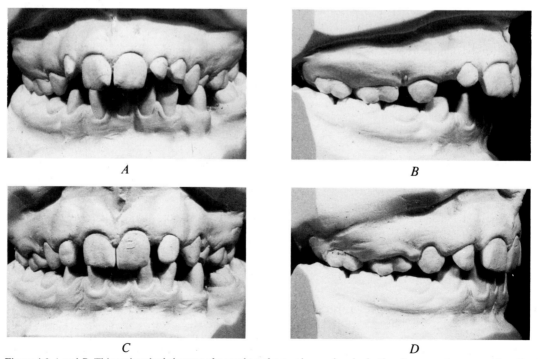

Figure 4.2 *A* and *B*, This patient had absence of a number of premolars and sucked a thumb, so creating an overjet; *C* and *D*, the incisors were retroclined and the lateral incisors were positioned in the centre of the space preparatory to crowning

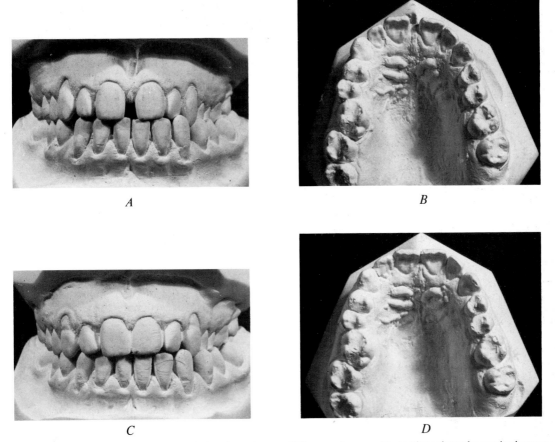

Figure 4.3 *A* and *B*, These are records of a female patient aged 30 years who was self-conscious about the spacing between the central incisors. There was also a tendency to prenormal occlusion and a reduced overbite. The fraenum labii was a well-defined Type 2; *C* and *D*, fraenectomy was performed and the central incisors approximated. The lateral incisors were moved mesially into contact with the centrals and spacing among the anterior teeth disappeared completely

welded to the bridge of a clasp on a tooth farther back in the arch (*Figure 4.6*). The welding must be done accurately and it is sensible to place a safety ligature as shown just in case the wire fractures if the appliance is roughly handled and the part above the weld becomes detached. The effect of the stabilizer is to restrict vertical movement without noticeably affecting the anteroposterior flexibility of the spring. The spring can then be applied to the tooth with great accuracy.

Mesiodistal movement of premolars and molars

Premolars and molars can be moved mesiodistally without difficulty using springs of 0.5 mm thickness. It is necessary to make the springs with a suitable combination of coil size and arm length. If the coil is too large and the arm too long, the spring may not generate enough pressure and prove difficult to keep in contact with the proper spot on the tooth. Again, the point at which the spring is fixed in relation to the tooth is important if the correct line of action is to be achieved (*Figure 4.7*).

When moving premolars distally into the space created by the removal of the first molar, it is perfectly feasible to move the two premolars with one spring. The practice of using separate springs for the premolars on the same side is to be deprecated as the appliance is unduly complicated for the patient, the spring for the second premolar is liable to become jammed between the teeth and it is inefficient to use two springs where one will suffice. Another practice which must be condemned is that of boxing-in springs if this is not necessary and can

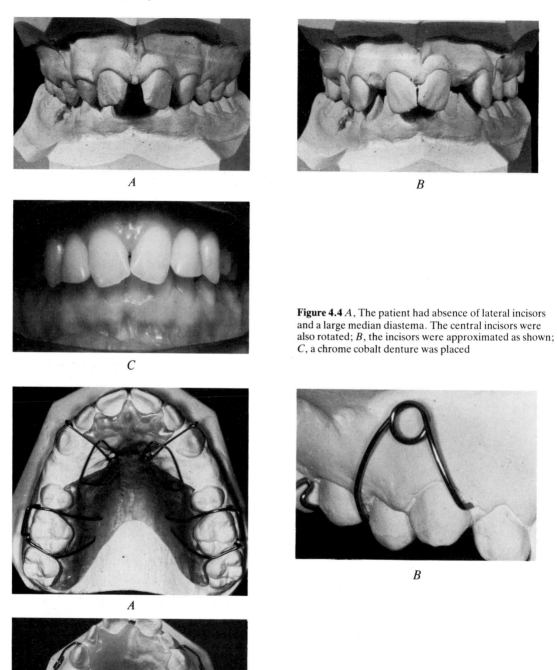

A

B

C

Figure 4.4 *A*, The patient had absence of lateral incisors and a large median diastema. The central incisors were also rotated; *B*, the incisors were approximated as shown; *C*, a chrome cobalt denture was placed

A

B

C

Figure 4.5 *A*, Palatal canine retractor springs. It is important with these springs to have the point of attachment sufficiently far forwards to ensure that the spring acts along the line of the dental arch; *B*, the standard buccal canine retractor; *C*, palatal view. The first premolars have not yet been removed. Note the distribution of the baseplate to gain maximum anchorage

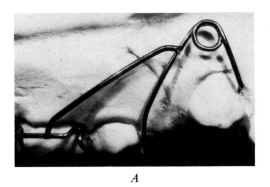

A

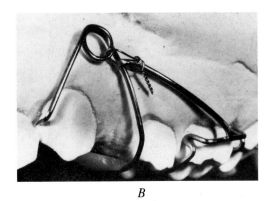

B

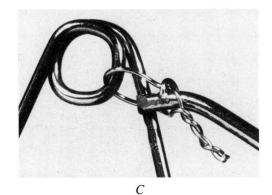

C

Figure 4.6 The stabilized canine retractor; *A*, the stabilizer is welded as shown to the spring and to the bridge of a molar clasp; *B* and *C*, the stabilized buccal canine retractor with safety ligature. The ligature runs through a little stirrup of soft 0.3 mm wire welded to the stabilizer and through the loop of the spring. If the canine retractor fractures due to rough handling of the appliance, the fracture usually occurs above the stabilizer and the ligature retains the loose piece

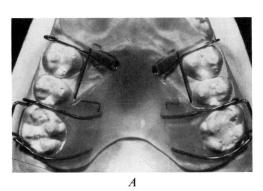

A

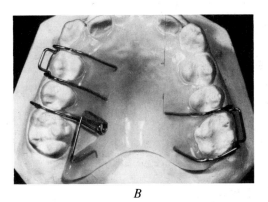

B

Figure 4.7 Palatal retractors for premolars and molars; *A*, the second premolar has not been removed; *B*, the molar is to be moved distally to provide room farther forwards

be avoided. Such boxing makes adjustments of the spring and guide unnecessarily difficult and is unhygienic. In some situations, making the baseplate continuous over springs is necessary to make the baseplate strong enough and the consequent disadvantages have to be accepted.

In the case shown in *Figure 4.8*, all the space for the permanent canines was obtained by moving the premolars distally into the spaces left by extraction of the first permanent molars due to severe caries. Anchorage was by clasping the second molars and using a Sved bite-plane.

The free ends of a palatal finger spring should be turned into a large loop (*Figure 4.9A*). This end then may be allowed to project a little which makes it easier for the patient to place the spring in position

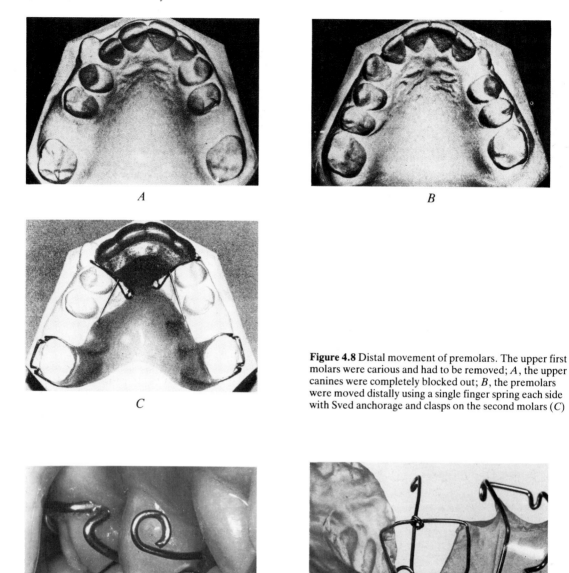

A

B

C

Figure 4.8 Distal movement of premolars. The upper first molars were carious and had to be removed; *A*, the upper canines were completely blocked out; *B*, the premolars were moved distally using a single finger spring each side with Sved anchorage and clasps on the second molars (*C*)

A

B

Figure 4.9 *A*, The free end of a palatal finger spring should be turned into a large loop as this will not injure the inside of the cheek. As shown, the loop can be quite large; *B*, the link which stabilizes the spring against the guide wire

and the smooth end will not injure the lip or cheek. A cut end, on the other hand, is uncomfortable and inconvenient and difficult for the patient to handle without risk of hurting the finger.

An important aid in the design of finger springs which run along wire guides is to link the spring to the guide wire with a loop of hard fine wire (*Figure 4.9B*). A hard wire of 0.3 mm thickness is wound twice tightly round the crossing and cut off closely. A probe is then pushed through the loop to open it sufficiently to let the spring move freely. The loop should be wound in the direction that allows the spring to run freely as it acts and not in the direction that causes the spring to jam as it acts.

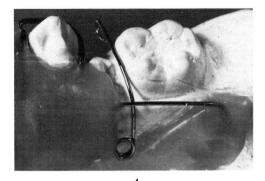

A

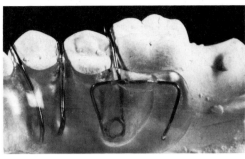

B

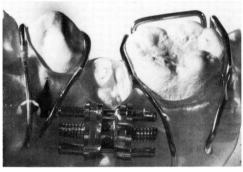

C

Figure 4.10 *A*, Distal movement of a lower molar. The spring lies in the lingual sulcus and the limb turns horizontally to lie in front of the molar; *B*, these springs of necessity need to be boxed in order to ensure that the baseplate is adequately strong; *C*, distal movement of a lower molar by means of a screw

The effect of such a link is to prevent the patient from accidentally lifting the spring away from the baseplate and so causing it to press into the gum and periodontal membrane. The spring also remains more accurately at its point of application and does not wander up and down the surface of the tooth that is being pressed on.

The lower arch

In the lower arch, a slight problem arises in that the plane of the spring and its coil are vertical but the arm must turn horizontally to lie against the approximal surface of the tooth to be moved. The answer is to make the spring neatly and the baseplate to fit accurately so that the patient will have as little inconvenience as possible. It is here that boxing in of the spring has to be accepted in order to make the baseplate strong enough (*Figure 4.10A* and *B*). Some mesiodistal movements may conveniently be done with screws. The distal movement of upper and lower molars is shown in *Figures 4.10C, 4.11* and *4.12*.

Lower canines can be moved mesiodistally by a buccal self-supporting spring in the same way as upper canines. It is not usually necessary to stabilize these springs in the lower arch as in the upper, although there is no reason why this should not be done if desired.

The lower incisors can be moved mesiodistally with removable appliances, but this movement is usually more expeditiously and efficiently carried out by means of multiband appliances which ensure complete control of the tooth arrangement, including rotations.

Disimpaction of molars

A special case of mesiodistal movement is the disimpaction of molar teeth which become impacted below the tooth immediately in front. This can happen to a first molar caught below the distal surface of the second deciduous molar or a second molar impacted below the first molar. This can occur both in the upper and in the lower arch (*Figure 4.13A–C*). Such impacted teeth can be freed by the use of a short spring of 0.9 mm wire as shown

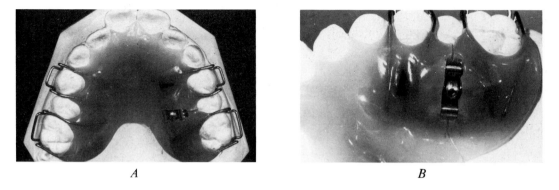

Figure 4.11 Distal movement of an upper molar by means of a screw; *A*, the general layout of the baseplate to gain maximum anchorage; *B*, the fitting of the screw

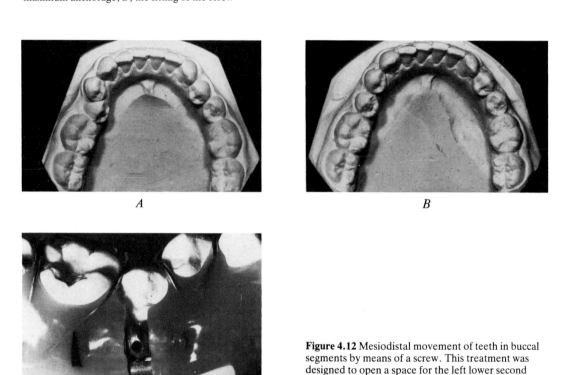

Figure 4.12 Mesiodistal movement of teeth in buccal segments by means of a screw. This treatment was designed to open a space for the left lower second premolar by reciprocal movement of the teeth in front of and behind this premolar; *A*, before treatment; *B*, after treatment; *C*, detail of the fitting of the screw

in *Figure 4.13D–F*. A spring of this kind is self-supporting, needing no guide or guard, and its range of action is very small. The end of the spring is flattened so that it can be placed exactly at the mesial surface of the semi-erupted tooth. When correctly constructed, the spring finds its way to the point of application and slips down the slope of the mesiolingual cusp of the tooth. Disimpaction only

requires a small movement which takes place in a few weeks and the appliance can be inspected at fortnightly intervals, if desired, in order to keep up adjustments which need to be of a very small amount (*Figure 4.13G* and *H*). An appliance of this kind can be used in the lower as well as in the upper arch.

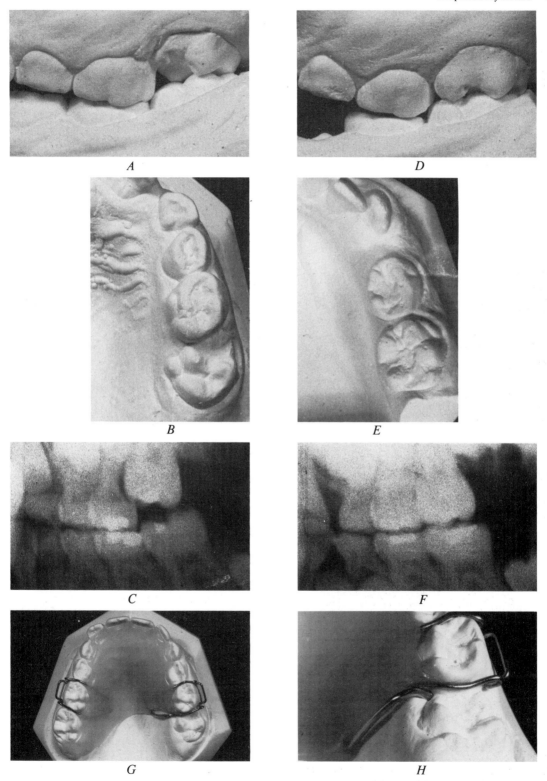

Figure 4.13 Disimpaction of the upper left first molar which is caught below the second deciduous molar; *A–C*, appearance before treatment; *D–F*, after treatment which took three months; *G* and *H*, the design of the appliance. Note the short, stiff spring which slips down mesially to the first molar. The activation of this spring is very slight, 0.5–1.0 mm, and the spring seats itself automatically when the appliance is inserted. Note also the clasp on the left upper second deciduous molar which ensures accurate retention of the appliance

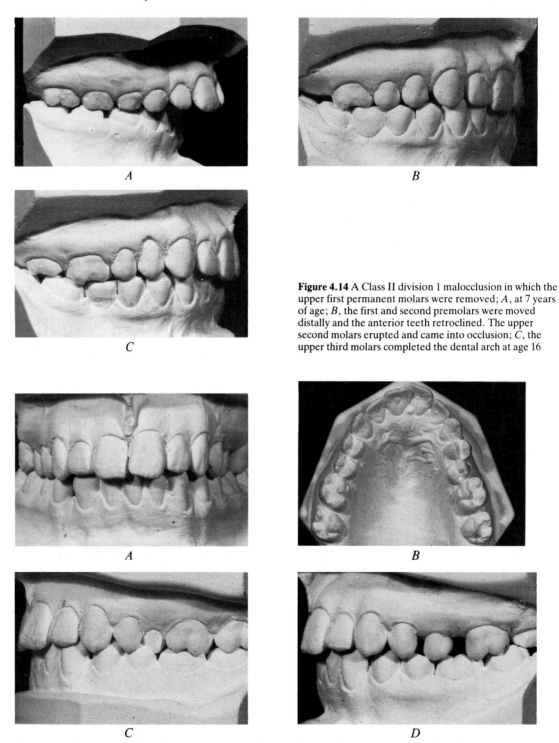

A

B

C

Figure 4.14 A Class II division 1 malocclusion in which the upper first permanent molars were removed; *A*, at 7 years of age; *B*, the first and second premolars were moved distally and the anterior teeth retroclined. The upper second molars erupted and came into occlusion; *C*, the upper third molars completed the dental arch at age 16

A

B

C

D

Figure 4.15 *A–C*, A patient aged 19 years complained of irregularity of the left upper central incisor. The upper third molars were as yet unerupted and there was crowding and impaction of the left upper second premolar; *D–H*, the upper second molars were extracted and the upper left first molar moved distally (*D* and *E*) followed by the first and second premolars and the canine (*F–H*). This made space for the left upper central and lateral incisors. The third molars erupted and made good contact with the first molars. The upper left central incisor was then rotated distolabially (*I* and *J*), and pericision done to help to stabilize the result; *K–M* show the appliances used to perform the distal movement of the left upper first molar, premolars and canine

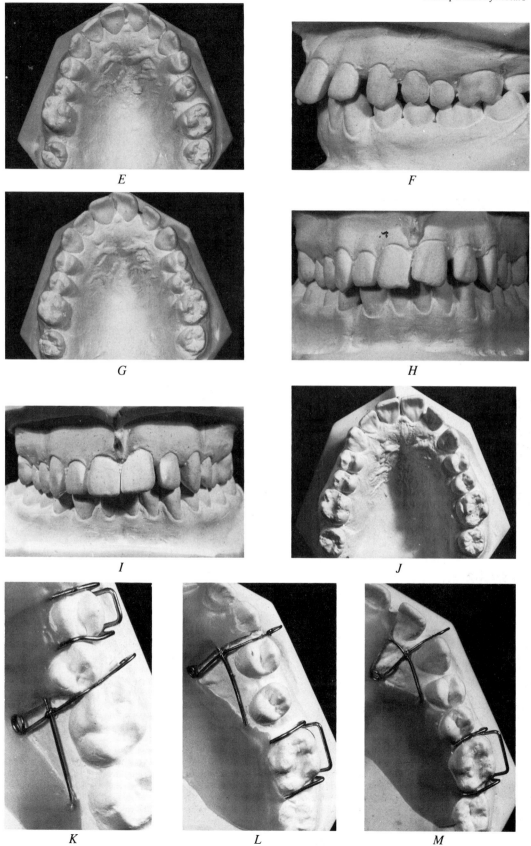

E

F

G

H

I

J

K

L

M

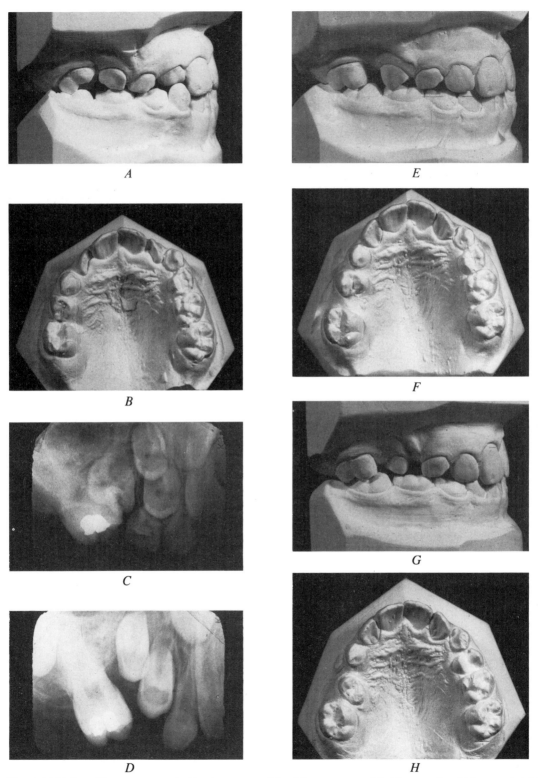

Figure 4.16 A boy of 9 years presented with submergence of the right upper second deciduous molar which was not visible in the mouth and the first and second premolars had not erupted. The right upper first permanent molar had inclined forward and there was about 1.0 mm of space between it and the first deciduous molar; *A–C*, clinical and X-ray appearances on first examination; *D*, the first and second deciduous molars have been removed; *E* and *F*, the first molar has been moved distally and retained in position and the first premolar has erupted; *G* and *H*, the first premolar has been removed and the second premolar has erupted

Case reports

Figure 4.14 shows the result of moving upper premolars distally after extracting upper first molars because of their carious condition. Space was thereby created for correction of a considerable overjet.

The subject shown in *Figure 4.15*, aged 19 years, complained of irregularity of the left upper central incisor which was worsening. Upper third molars were approaching eruption. The upper second molars were removed and the space of the left upper second molar was transferred to the region of the upper left incisors by distal movement of the left upper canine, premolars and first molar. The third molars erupted and made good contact with the first molars.

The boy of 9 years whose records are shown in *Figure 4.16* presented with the right upper second deciduous molar submerged and out of sight. The first permanent molar was severely tilted and almost in contact with the first deciduous molar. There was an underlying crowding of the dentition (Angle Class I). The right upper first and second deciduous molars were removed and the first permanent molar was moved distally. The first premolar thereafter erupted and was removed. The second premolar then erupted. The patient, now aged 13, was very slow in getting teeth. It was anticipated that removal of three further permanent units would be needed in connection with orthodontic treatment.

Chapter 5

Rotation and root movement of teeth

There are certain rotation and root movements that removable appliances can perform very well and it is helpful to bear these possibilities in mind when considering treatment problems.

The production of a rotary movement requires the application of two equal and opposite pressures acting at a distance apart to produce a mechanical couple (*see Figure 2.19A*). This will produce rotation about a point somewhere between the lines of action of the two forces. It is therefore necessary to find, on a tooth to be rotated, two points at a suitable distance apart on which pressures in opposite directions may be applied, and this requirement automatically eliminates the possibility of rotating certain teeth. For instance, canines, upper and lower, are of a rounded shape which does

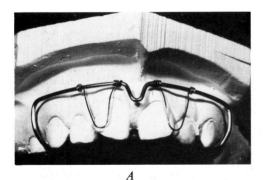

A

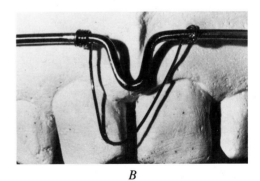

B

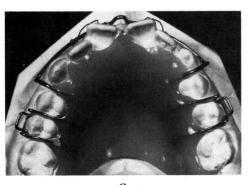

C

Figure 5.1 Apron springs on high labial arches which apply precise pressure on the corners and edges of the incisor teeth; *A*, pressure on distal corners of the upper central incisors; *B*, pressure on a single central incisor; *C*, lingual view of *A*

not offer two points near the outside of the contour of the tooth to which suitable pressures may be applied. Lower incisors, again, are so small in width that the forces even when applied at the extreme ends of the incisal edge are so close together that an effective mechanical couple cannot be produced.

It is important when constructing appliances for rotation and root movement to ensure that the springs act exactly at the points intended and do not slide away to some other nearby but unsuitable point. For this reason it is sometimes necessary to make springs rather stiff in order to ensure accuracy of application to the teeth and to accept the short range of action inherent in such springs. Cantilever springs are perfectly suitable for developing the necessary pressures. On the labial side, accurately made apron springs supported on a high labial arch are effective (*Figure 5.1*), or self-supporting springs of 0.7 mm wire may be used (*Figure 5.2*). On the lingual side, cantilever springs may be used (*Figure 5.3*), or the torque spring is flexible but at the same time robust (*Figure 5.4*).

The torque spring and self-supporting labial spring are a useful combination and can be used effectively for single teeth.

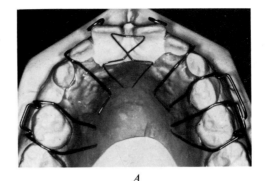

A

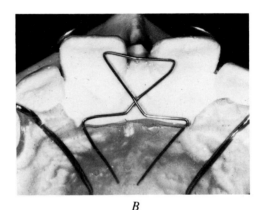

B

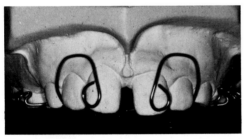

Figure 5.2 Self-supporting springs placed at the distal edges of incisor teeth

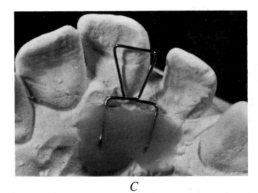

C

Figure 5.4 The torque spring used to apply pressure from the lingual aspect to produce rotation; *A* and *B*, a double spring acting on two teeth; *C*, a single torque spring

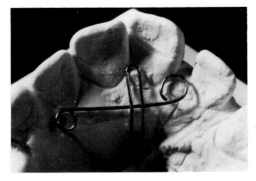

Figure 5.3 The lingual cantilever spring designed to apply pressure precisely to the edge of an incisor tooth to produce one component of a mechanical couple

Rotation of upper incisors

Possibilities for the use of these appliances are shown in *Figures 5.5, 5.6, 5.7* and *5.8*. If the lateral incisors are wide enough, they can be rotated with such removable appliances.

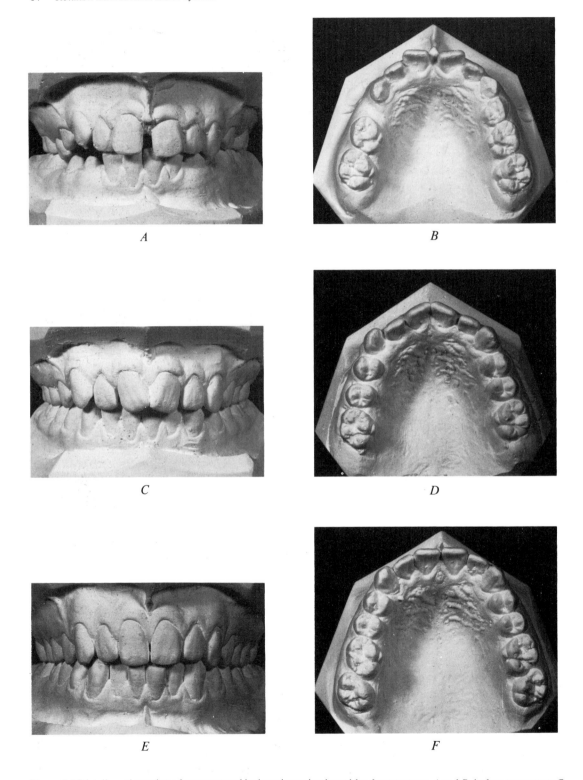

Figure 5.5 Distolingual rotation of upper central incisors in conjuction with a fraenectomy; *A* and *B*, before treatment; *C* and *D*, showing over-rotation of the central incisors; *E* and *F*, the teeth have settled into correct alignment

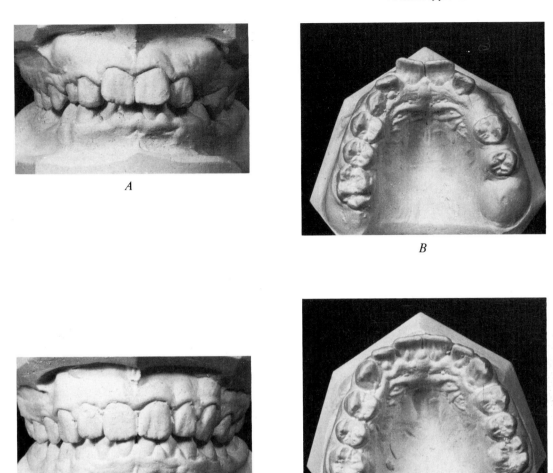

Figure 5.6 Distolingual rotation of central incisors. In this patient, oral hygiene was not good and the first molars were removed as part of orthodontic treatment; *A* and *B*, before treatment; *C* and *D*, at end of treatment

Rotation of premolars and molars

A common misplacement of the upper first premolar is to find the lingual cusp rotated mesially and biting buccally to the lower first premolar (*Figure 5.9A* and *B*). Rotation of the upper premolar by swinging the lingual cusp distally will produce correct occlusion (*Figure 5.9C* and *D*). This rotation may be performed by pressing firmly on the mesial surface of the tooth opposite the lingual cusp. The buccal cusp rests against the mesial surface of the tooth behind and the tooth rotates about its point of contact with the second premolar (*Figure 5.10A* and *B*). It will be noticed that here only one force is used

and that the place of the second is taken by a fixed point, the point of contact, between the first and second premolars. There is, therefore, in this case not strictly a couple but a force rotating about a point. The value of the force for rotation purposes is given by the moment of the force about this point. As the distance between the line of action of the force and the point is comparatively small, the value of this moment is low, hence the rotating effort is small. It is found clinically that rotations such as this take a considerable time.

Another common tooth misplacement is the mesiolingual rotation of the upper first permanent molar, which considerably reduces the space re-

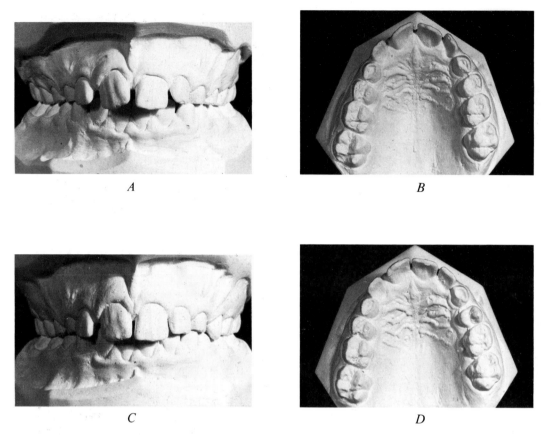

Figure 5.7 *A* and *B*, A patient aged 8 years with rotation of the upper central and lateral incisors; *C* and *D*, the teeth were aligned with self-supporting springs on the labial side and torque springs on the lingual side

quired for the second premolar (*Figure 5.11A*). The molar tooth may be rotated distally by pressure on the mesial surface opposite to the mesiobuccal cusp (*Figure 5.11B*). Rotation takes place about the palatal root (*Figure 5.11C*).

Root movement

This term refers to the tipping of apices in one direction or the other, a movement that is usually performed with most of the fixed appliances. If it is desired to tilt the roots of an upper incisor mesially or distally, this may be done by applying equal and opposite pressures to the mesial and distal surfaces of the crown of the tooth near the incisal edge and at the cervical margin (*see Figure 2.19E*).

Figure 5.12A shows the palatal view of the two finger springs which press with equal and opposite pressures at the cervical margins of the central

incisors in a mesial direction. The incisors have been tipped together but are prevented from moving further mesially at the incisal edges by the stop wire of 0.7 mm stainless steel with a little T piece on the labial aspect of the teeth. This arrangement also prevents the teeth from overlapping under the pressure at the distal surfaces (*Figure 5.12B*). If this appliance is adjusted and worn carefully, the apices of the incisors will become tipped together (*Figure 5.13*). The patient shown in *Figure 5.13* was aged 17 years and had excellent occlusion apart from absence of the permanent upper lateral incisors. The central incisors had spaced out as shown but the rest of the dental arch showed interproximal contact between the teeth.

The lingual tipping of upper anterior tooth roots is a movement which is usually thought of in connection with fixed multiband appliances. Bass (1975) has shown that it is possible to perform this movement by pressure in a lingual direction at the

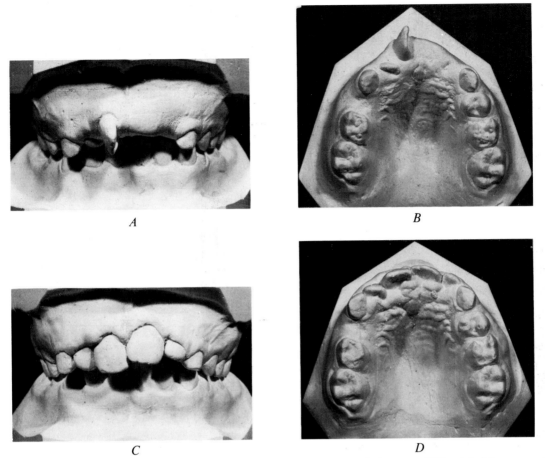

A

B

C

D

Figure 5.8 A patient aged 8.5 years who presented with the right upper central incisor rotated 90° and the left upper central unerupted. The unerupted tooth was exposed and erupted satisfactorily. The right central was rotated with a removable appliance and the two incisors remained in good alignment. The patient had an underlying postnormal occlusion which was eventually treated by conventinonal means; *A* and *B*, before treatment; *C* and *D*, at the end of treatment

gingival margin on the incisors while preventing lingual movement at the incisal edges by using a Sved bite-plane (*see Figure 2.19F*).

An appliance for this purpose is illustrated in *Figure 5.14*. Clasps should be placed well forwards to ensure accurate fitting of the Sved bite-plane and it is as well to clasp the first molar teeth also. The spring shown acts on both incisors but separate springs may be placed on each tooth. The spring is really a double-ended cantilever of 0.6 mm wire and its short length and small coils render it fairly strong in action. In practice only a short activation is given and as a bodily movement is being effected, fairly firm pressure can be used. Tubes may be soldered to the first premolar clasps and extra-oral traction may be used to reinforce anchorage at night time.

The baseplate must be left thick enough behind the incisors so that it can be cut away to allow the teeth to tilt lingually at the apices.

Teeth which do not present points at which pressures may be applied to produce rotatory movements may be rotated and tipped by means of a whip spring locked into an attachment banded or bonded to the tooth.

A box-type of attachment was used by Watkin (1933) for his modification of the pin-and-tube appliance and a box attachment in stainless steel was described by Friel and McKeag (1939) (*Figure 5.15*). This box was well known as the 'McKeag box'.

The McKeag box has been used for not only the Watkin pin-and-tube appliance, but also for the whip spring to develop tipping and rotatory moments on single teeth.

The McKeag box was, for many years, available

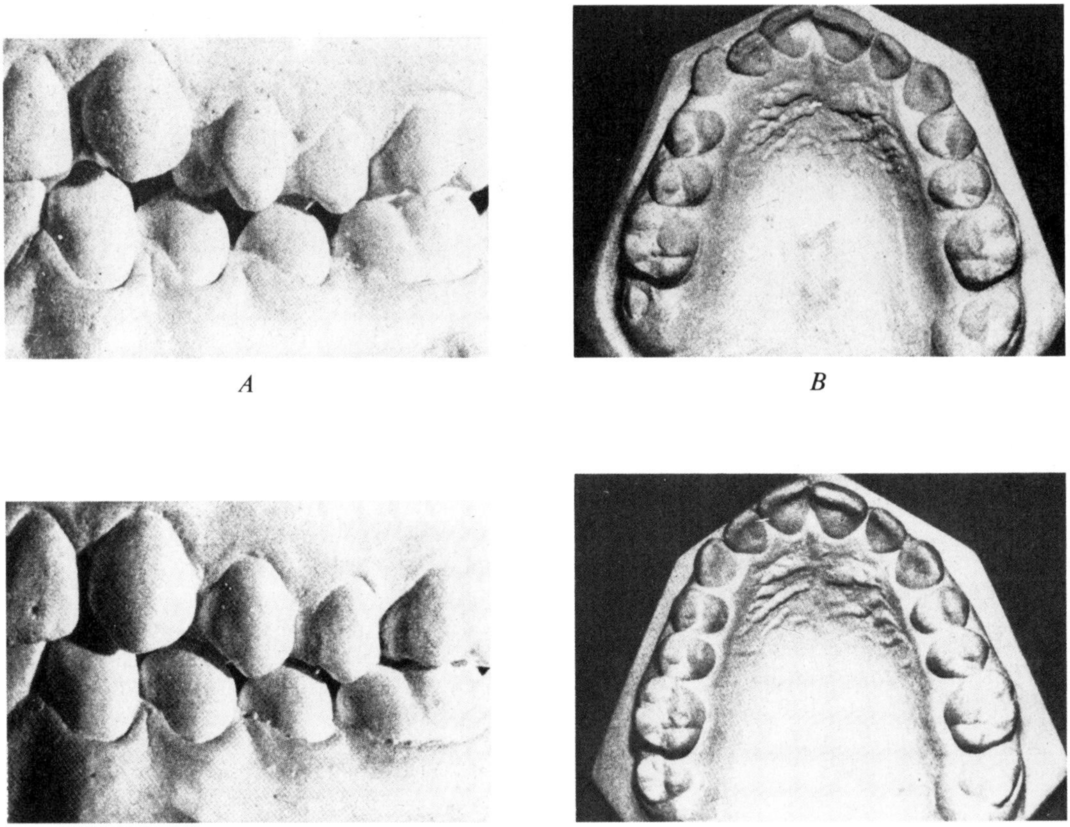

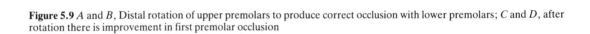

A   *B*

C   *D*

Figure 5.9 *A* and *B*, Distal rotation of upper premolars to produce correct occlusion with lower premolars; *C* and *D*, after rotation there is improvement in first premolar occlusion

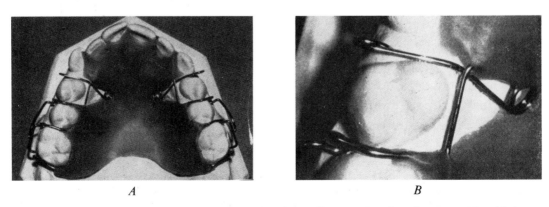

A   *B*

Figure 5.10 *A*, The appliance used to produce distal rotation of upper first premolars about the contact point with the second premolars; *B*, the point of application of pressure on the first premolar

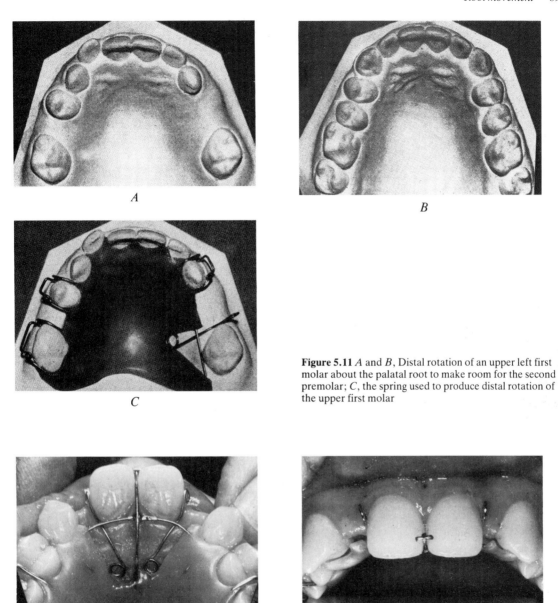

Figure 5.11 *A* and *B*, Distal rotation of an upper left first molar about the palatal root to make room for the second premolar; *C*, the spring used to produce distal rotation of the upper first molar

Figure 5.12 The mesial tipping of the apices of upper central incisors; *A*, a stop and restraining piece have been put near the incisal edges between the central incisors; *B*, the finger springs act at the gum margins

commercially and presses and pliers could also be procured or were made up by practitioners for the fabrication of the device as required. There has, however, been a move towards currently available precision attachments which are sometimes pressed into service for use with the whip spring. Being designed for attachment to an archwire that passes through, however, it is not always a simple matter to fix a whip spring firmly enough to eliminate lost motion in the attachment. The Minibox, however, is a simple and effective successor to the McKeag box and brings the advantages of compactness and greater strength and the fact that no equipment is needed for its production.

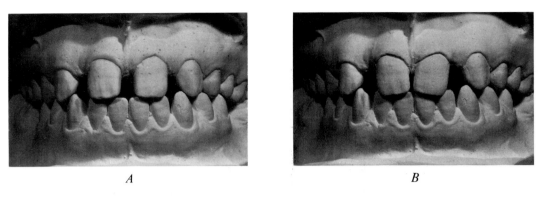

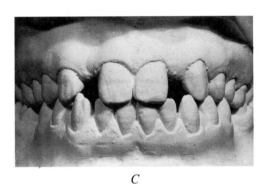

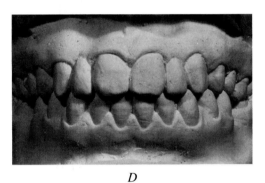

Figure 5.13 Upper central incisor space closure and root alignment in a patient aged 17 years; *A*, before treatment; *B*, the incisors have been inclined together; *C*, the apices have been tipped mesially; *D*, a prosthesis has been fitted

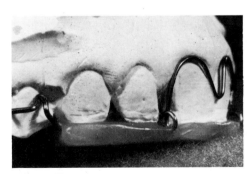

Figure 5.14 Lingual root torque on upper incisors. A Sved plate is used and pressure in a lingual direction is applied by a special double-ended cantilever spring as shown or separate springs may be used on each tooth

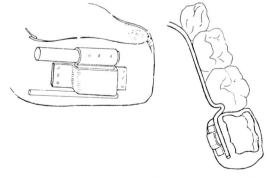

Figure 5.15 The McKeag box. This box accepts a post 3 × 0.6 mm in size. The box is pressed from strip and welded by a flange at each end. Introduced originally for lingual arches of 1.0 mm wire

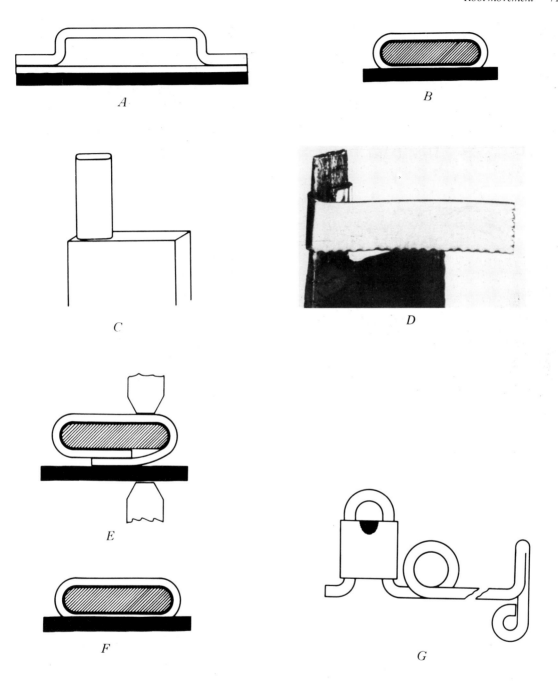

Figure 5.16. The construction of the Minibox; *A* and *B*, comparison of a cross-section of the Minibox, *B*, with the McKeag box, *A*. The Minibox is narrower and flatter than the McKeag box and is made for posts 2.5 mm × 0.5 mm in size; *C* and *D*, the Minibox is made by wrapping band material 0.15 mm thick and 3.0 mm wide round a former of copper. The former is filed from copper strip and is made 0.5 mm thick, 2.5 mm wide and about 4.0 mm long. The edges are rounded. Band material is wrapped round the former *D*, and cut off and flattened; *E* and *F*, welding the Minibox. The box is welded right through to the band or backing. The copper former conducts the current but does not weld to the steel. The box is then pressed off the former; *G* and *H*, the whip spring is made of 0.5 or 0.4 mm wire and held in the box by a slight dent at the top edge. The spring is removed by pinching the curve of the post against the bottom edge of the box with spring forming pliers

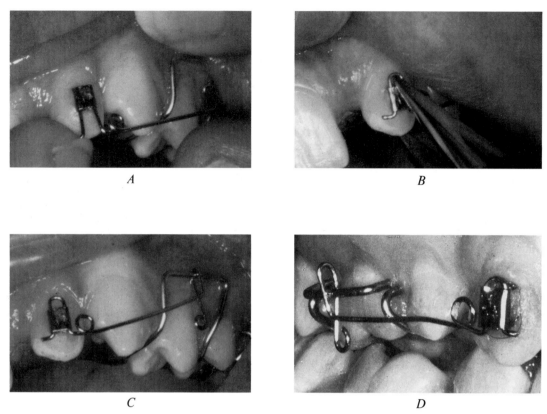

Figure 5.17 The Minibox in use; *A*, placing the whip spring in position; *B*, denting the top edge of the box for retention of the post; *C*, the whip spring hooked onto a special wire support on the baseplate; *D*, the whip spring used for rotation of a canine tooth

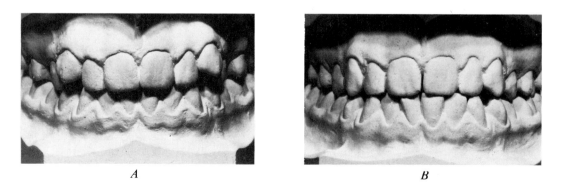

Figure 5.18 Rotation and distal root tipping of upper canines; *A*, before treatment; *B*, after treatment

Figure 5.16A shows that the McKeag box is pressed from strip stainless steel with a flange at either end for welding to a band and, today, to a backing for bonding purposes. The standard box is made for a post 3.0 mm wide and 0.6 mm thick. The flanges and thickness of the material of the box make a total width for the attachment of about 5.0 mm. When welded to a band or bonded to a tooth, especially a small tooth, such an attachment is unduly bulky and difficult to fit to the contour of an anterior tooth in particular. Also the attachment is made for too thick a post as the preferred wire for a whip arch is 0.5 or 0.4 mm.

The Minibox, however, does not have flanges but is wrapped around the post, in this case a U loop, and is welded directly to the band or to the backing, without flanges (*Figure 5.16B*).

The construction of the box is of the utmost simplicity. *Figure 5.16C* shows a strip of copper with a post filed at one end. The post measures 0.5 mm thick and about 2.5 mm wide and is filed using a fine jeweller's file. The post should be about 4.0 mm long.

To make a Minibox, band material of 0.15 mm thickness is wrapped round the copper post using Howe pliers, and the excess cut off (*Figure 5.16D*). The Minibox is then welded to a band or to a gauze backing (*Figure 5.16E*). The copper post conducts the welding current but does not weld to the steel band material. The box is then carefully pressed and rocked off the post and the backing trimmed to the size of the box (*Figure 5.16F*).

The post of the spring is a U loop which should be made to fit the box with a little tension to ensure absence of 'slop' or lost motion.

The whip arch fits as shown in *Figure 5.16G* and *H* and the spring is locked into the box by slightly denting the top edge. A slight dent only is needed. The box should not be flattened in or else the post will be very difficult to remove. To remove the post, the curve of the U is pinched against the bottom edge of the box with spring-forming pliers when the post will snap past the dent in the top edge. The post is then gently rocked out of the box. The free end of the whip spring is looped onto the bridge of a clasp or a loop of wire can be placed in the buccal sulcus especially for the purpose.

The appliance is shown in use in *Figure 5.17*. With this attachment, teeth may be rotated and tipped as required using a molar clasp or a loop of wire placed a short distance away in the buccal sulcus. It is also possible to hook a whip spring onto a labial bow where the direction of rotation requires an attachment towards the front.

Figure 5.18 shows the correction of rotated upper canine teeth.

Chapter 6

Expansion/contraction

Orthodontic expansion of the dental arches has long been a subject of controversy. There is still debate as to whether arch width and size are determined by facial build or by the moulding activity of the soft tissues of the face and mouth. A factor broadly known as the compensatory capacity of the alveolar structures to carry the teeth into satisfactory arch form has been suggested and breakdown of this factor is brought forward as the cause of unsatisfactory tooth arrangement which must include, in some cases, lack of width of the arch form.

There is no problem regarding arch width if the occlusal relationship is correct buccolingually and the form of both the individual arches is a smooth harmonious curve.

Today it is generally agreed that expansion of both upper and lower dental arches simultaneously is not a satisfactory procedure in view of the inevitable relapse that occurs to an unpredictable degree. It is sometimes maintained that rapid and extensive lateral expansion, particularly of the upper arch and involving separation of the mid-palatal suture, can be used to produce a permanent widening of the dental arches because of what is termed 'controlled relapse' to a predicted dimension.

The whole procedure must be looked at from the point of view of what is being attempted. It is sometimes maintained that crowding of anterior teeth is attributable to lack of arch width and that lateral expansion will produce space for the correction of such crowding. Lateral expansion of the arches does not produce significant space for the correction of anterior crowding, and in crowding conditions alignment of the labial segments without extracting teeth at some point to create space produces a rounding out of the anterior teeth into a wider circle by means of proclination of these teeth.

Dental arch expansion, whether lateral or antero-posterior, tends to place segments of the dental arches in positions which are not stable and from which relapse of more or less degree will take place in the absence of some new stabilizing factor.

The main role of expansion is the possibility of correcting discrepancies of buccolingual occlusion by buccal or lingual movement of these segments as a whole by using expansion or contraction appliances.

It is here that the removable appliance is well fitted to operate and clasped expansion appliances can efficiently produce expansion or contraction of the buccal segments. It is important, however, to regard this movement as intended for the correction buccolingually of occlusal relationships rather than to gain space for anterior teeth by a general widening of the dental arch.

Anchorage problems do not as a rule arise, as expansion implies that simultaneous equal and opposite movements are being carried out. The force employed and its reaction are, therefore, both being made to do useful work.

Lateral expansion of the upper arch

Expansion of the upper arch can be carried out by means of a simple baseplate with a screw placed so as to act in a transverse direction (*Figure 6.1*). The screw should be placed midway between the most anterior point and the most posterior point on either side at which pressure is to be exerted. This is necessary so that, as far as possible, leverage on the screw is avoided. Leverage leads to the imposition of bending forces on the screw and in consequence the risk of a fracture.

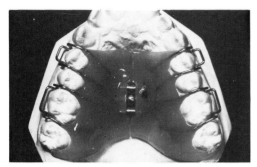

Figure 6.1 The upper expansion appliance, formerly known as the Badcock plate, in tribute to its originator. An equal amount of pressure is produced at either side of the appliance

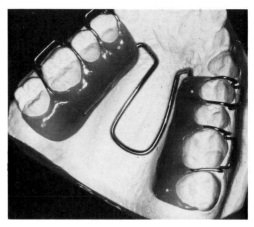

Figure 6.2 The upper expansion arch or Coffin spring, so named after its originator. The small registration pits can be seen anteriorly and posteriorly. The archwire is 1.25 mm thick

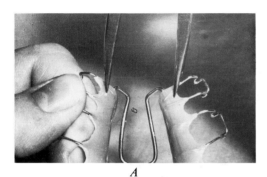

A

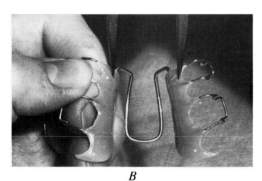

B

Figure 6.3 Registration of the expansion imparted to the upper expansion arch; *A*, before activation; *B*, after activation

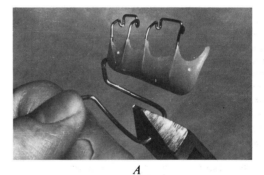

A

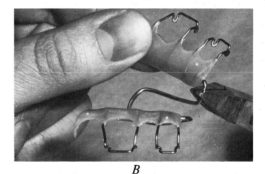

B

Figure 6.4 Adjustment of the upper expansion arch; *A*, slight straightening of the archwire at the spot grasped in the pliers produces an expansion at the anterior end of the appliance; *B*, adjustment for expansion at the posterior end for each side separately. The archwire is held firmly at the spot shown and the posterior end of the appliance is moved laterally in a horizontal plane. The other side is adjusted similarly

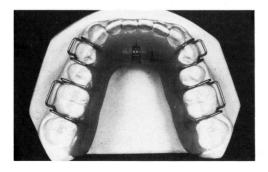

Figure 6.5 The lower expansion appliance or lower Badcock plate

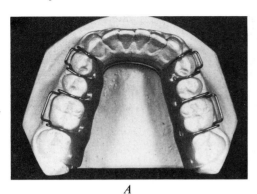
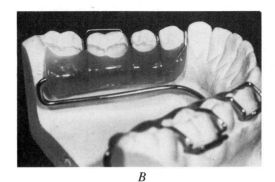

A   B

Figure 6.6 *A*, The lower expansion arch or Coffin spring; *B*, the disposition of the arch in the premolar and molar region

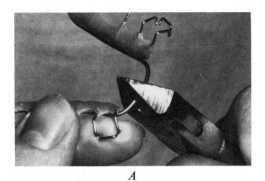
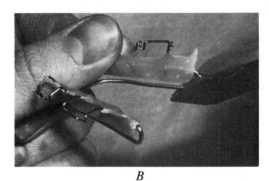

A   B

Figure 6.7 Adjustment of the lower expansion arch; *A*, for adjustment posteriorly the middle section of the arch is straightened slightly by grasping firmly with Adams Universal Pliers; *B*, the anterior ends are adjusted by grasping each posterior end firmly as shown and adjusting the anterior end in a horizontal direction. Registration of expansion is carried out as shown in *Figure 6.3*

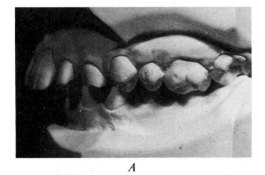
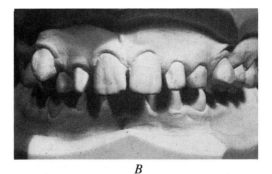

A   B

Figure 6.8 The patient is a boy aged 13 years; *A–D*, before treatment. The problem included a very large upper arch with a severe irregularity in the right upper canine region and non-eruption of the left upper canine tooth. Treatment included exposure of the canine and alignment of the upper arch. The arch relationship buccolingually was corrected by means of a lower expansion plate of the Coffin type; *E–H*, dental casts at age 18 years

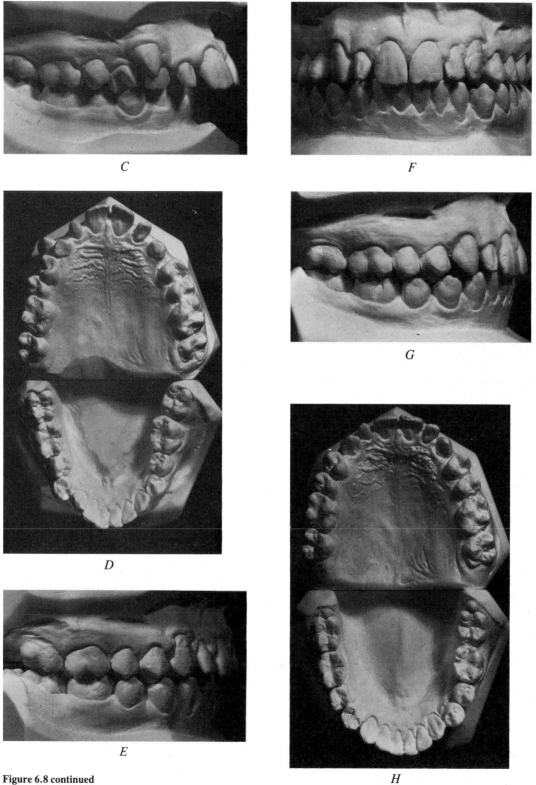

C

D

E

F

G

H

Figure 6.8 continued

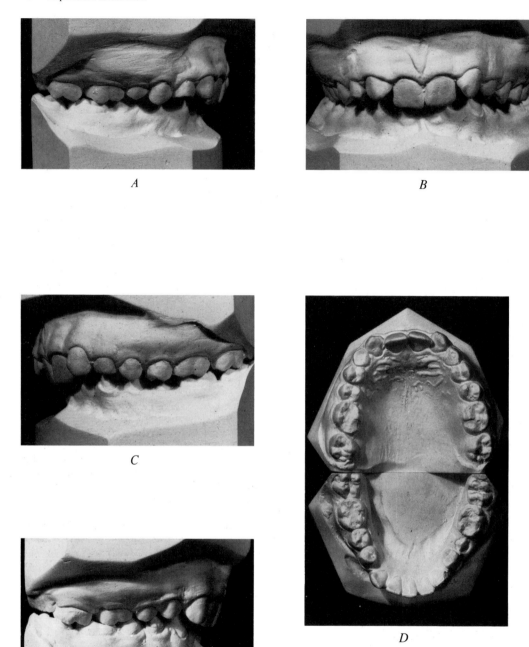

A

B

C

D

E

Figure 6.9 Patient aged 12 years with a well-arranged lower arch with spacing. The premolars are in scissors bite and the upper arches rather wide. Treatment entailed contraction of the upper arch using an appliance with clasps on first premolars and first molars and a bridge between the clasps to bring the second premolars lingually. Correct buccolingual occlusion was achieved and the lower arch was treated with a lower multiband to align the left lower second premolar. The upper lateral incisors are to be aligned and suitably adjusted in shape; *A–D*, before treatment; *E–H*, after treatment

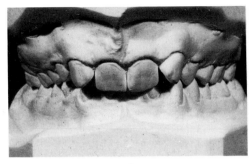

F

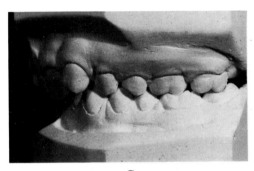

G

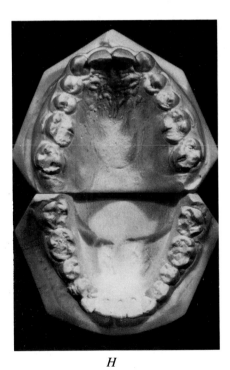

H

Figure 6.9 continued

If different degrees of expansion are required at the front and at the back of the buccal segments an expansion arch type of appliance should be used.

An appliance of this kind was described by Walter H. Coffin in 1881, and the arch or spring which produces the force or pressure is today commonly known as the Coffin spring after its originator.

Originally the baseplate was made in one piece and cut down the midline with a fine saw after vulcanizing. Present-day practice is to make the baseplate in two small segments, large enough to make contact with all the teeth to be moved and to contain the tags of the clasps and the ends of the archwire (*Figure 6.2*).

The archwire is of 1.25 mm thickness and is formed with a generous loop in the centre; it stands 1.0 mm away from the soft tissue of the palate. The archwire is usually made first and the tags of the clasps looped over it before constructing the baseplate. Four small pits should be drilled with a very fine rosehead bur, one at each extremity of the baseplate, and these are used as registration points for recording, by means of dividers, the amount of expansion or activity given to the appliance before it is inserted.

The amount of activation given to such an appliance before insertion will depend on the length and thickness of the archwire and on the number of teeth being moved. Experience shows, however, that a range of activity of 2.0 mm (1.0 mm each side) is usually sufficient at a time, and further degrees of expansion are achieved by subsequent adjustments.

Before any adjustment is made to an appliance of this kind the width between the registration point anteriorly and posteriorly should be measured with dividers and recorded. The amount of expansion given to the appliance will then be known (*Figure 6.3*).

Adjustment of the appliance is effected by grasping the centre of the arch with Adams Universal Pliers and squeezing firmly, when the anterior end of the appliance will expand (*Figure 6.4A*). Expansion of the posterior ends is done by opening the appliance at the back by adjustment at the anterior ends of the arch. It is necessary to make this adjustment by grasping a straight section of the arch in the pliers and bending the distal end of the appliance laterally (*Figure 6.4B*). Making the adjustment by grasping a bend in the arch at the front with the pliers and squeezing it will not do as the arch does not run horizontally in this section and making the adjustment in this way will tip the distal end of the appliance away from the palate as well as laterally. If both ends of the appliance are adjusted in this way and hence tipped, the effect will be to tip the loop of the arch into the palate. Making an adjustment at the anterior ends of the appliance by squeezing the archwire only is very likely to introduce warpage and distortion.

Lateral expansion of the lower arch

Lateral expansion of the lower arch can be effected with a screw type of appliance with the screw placed in the middle line behind the incisors (*Figure 6.5*). With this arrangement, however, leverage on the screw is very great and any bending of the screw will result in lack of expansion at the distal parts of the arch.

A better arrangement is to use the Coffin spring or expansion arch type of appliance. Not only is this appliance efficient but an easily controlled difference in expansion can be produced anteriorly or posteriorly as may be desired (*Figure 6.6*).

As with the upper arch expansion appliance, the baseplate is only large enough to contain the ends of the arch and the tags of the clasps. The arch is 1.25 mm thick and registration pits are made at the ends of the baseplate. Adjustment of the appliance is done in much the same way as for the upper type of appliance. The posterior ends of the appliance are expanded by grasping the curved horizontal middle section of the arch with Adams Universal Pliers (*Figure 6.7A*) and squeezing firmly and precisely.

Adjustment of the anterior ends is made for each side separately while gripping the distal ends of the arch firmly by a section that cannot be distorted by pressure of the pliers (*Figure 6.7B*). The range of activity should be about 2.0–4.0 mm at a time, further expansion being done by subsequent adjustment.

The cases shown in *Figures 6.8* and *6.9* illustrate the adjustment of the width of one arch to match the other. In *Figure 6.8* the lower arch was expanded to match the upper and in *Figure 6.9* the upper arch was contracted to match the lower.

Chapter 7

Intermaxillary and extra-oral traction

The design of traction plates does not differ greatly from that of ordinary upper or lower removable appliances. Firm retention for the appliances is necessary so that four clasps on each plate are normally required. Where four claspable teeth are not present use may be made of the accessory arrowhead clasp to increase retention of the appliance. It is not so much that the appliance requires to be fiercely clasped to the teeth but that it needs to be positively supported at each corner, so that levering and tipping effects are resisted.

The lower traction appliance

The standard lower traction appliance is clasped on the first premolars and first permanent molars (*Figure 7.1*). In some instances this retention is not available because the first premolar has not erupted. It is then necessary to put an auxiliary arrowhead clasp on a second deciduous molar. The lower traction hook on the first permanent molar may be of the standard type.

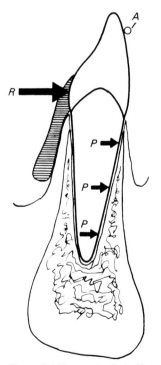

Figure 7.2 The mechanical effect of the labial bow in the lower traction plate. The reaction R transmitted through the baseplate tends to procline the lower incisors. The labial arch, A, prevents proclination and converts the pressure on the lower incisors into pressure P, P, P, distributed evenly over the labial alveolar bone. An element of 'stationary anchorage' is thereby created

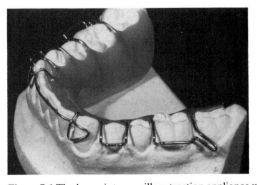

Figure 7.1 The lower intermaxillary traction appliance with clasps on four teeth, hooks on the molar clasps and labial bow. The hooks may be welded onto the clasps as an afterthought but the hooks shown are stronger. It is also possible to place a loop in the bridge of the molar clasp to act as a hook

An indispensable feature of the lower traction plate is the labial bow (*Figure 7.2*). This bow serves the purpose of preventing proclination of the lower incisors. The bow must lie accurately against the labial surfaces of the incisors and canines nearly at their incisal edge. These teeth are thus prevented from inclining forwards under the pressure exerted on them from behind and so become more resistant to movement than if they are simply permitted to tilt forwards. An element of 'stationary anchorage' is therefore obtained.

As the embrasures between the canines and the first premolars are already occupied by the wire of the premolar clasp, the tags of the bow are brought lingually between the canines and the lateral incisors. The wire used for the bow should be 0.6 mm.

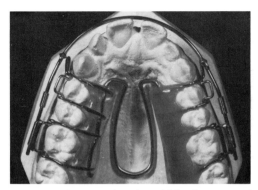

Figure 7.4 Upper traction plate with hooks on premolar clasps. Coffin spring and free-sliding labial bow with stop hooks

Upper traction appliances

Upper traction appliances consist of baseplates clasped to the first premolars and first molars and provided with a means of expanding the baseplates in a lateral direction (*Figure 7.3*). This expansion mechanism is not necessarily provided for actively expanding the arch but is to permit expansion of the plate following the distal movement of the upper buccal segments. Distal movement is accompanied by expansion, because the teeth in moving distally move to a wider part of the arch. The expansion mechanism may be either the conventional screw or the Coffin expansion arch (*Figure 7.4*).

The standard traction plate, clasped to the first premolars and first molars, is designed to produce distal movement of the buccal segments only. By dividing the operation of moving the upper arch distally into two stages, moving the buccal segments distally first, then retracting the upper incisors and canines separately, strain on the anchorage of the lower arch can be reduced.

When the upper buccal segments have been retracted and it is desired to retract the incisors and

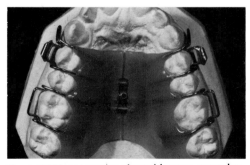

Figure 7.3 Upper traction plate with screw, premolar hooks and tubes on premolar clasps

canines, a free-sliding labial arch may be added to the upper appliance running in tubes soldered to the molar clasps. These tubes may be placed on the clasps from the outset in anticipation of the second phase of treatment or they may easily be added later when required.

It is necessary to make the free-sliding arch of wire 0.9 mm thick to match the archwire with the tubing in order to ensure that the arch runs freely in the tubes.

The traction hook on the buccal arch (*Figure 7.5A*), is also a stop for extra-oral traction. It is made from 0.7 mm soft stainless steel wire, welded or soldered, and turned round the archwire. The free end is then turned backwards into a hook as shown.

Extra-oral traction

Extra-oral traction makes use of the anchorage of the back of the head and neck through the use of headgear. Headgear consists of a headcap or collar which distributes the reaction to the head or neck and contains the elastic element which stores the energy or force which is conveyed to the teeth.

Headcaps are open-work harnesses, formerly of leather or fabric, but today made of plastic products resembling one or other of these materials or with a smooth, hygienic surface. Cervical attachments are simple collars or straps to which are attached or in which are contained the elastic components.

Numerous variations of these devices are made commercially and recommended from time to time, each designed to make fitting and using easier and to overcome some particular difficulty.

Extra-oral headgear is connected to the intra-oral appliance in one of two ways. Either extensions of the intra-oral appliance are brought out at either

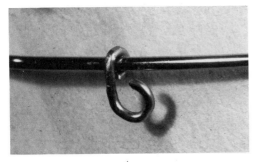

A

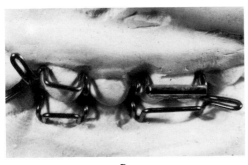

B

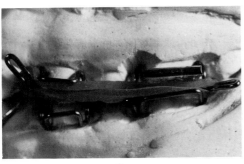

C

Figure 7.5 *A*, The stop hook. This is placed on a free-sliding labial bow. It is made of 0.7 mm soft stainless steel wire welded or soldered to the bow and turned round it. The hook curls backwards and an extra-oral attachment can be hooked on in front (*see Figure 7.8D*); *B*, intermaxillary traction hooks on upper premolar and lower molar; *C*, intermaxillary elastic in place

side and elastics are looped onto them from the headgear, or else curved arms reach from the headgear into the mouth and hook onto the intra-oral appliance.

In the first arrangement, elastics are simply looped between the headgear and the extra-oral extensions or 'whiskers' as they are sometimes

called, and in the second, arrangements must be made to ensure that the curved arm is guided and supported in the headgear. This means that some tubular section forms part of the headgear.

Today, ready-made headgear and extra-oral attachments are available, complete with instructions for their use. It is, however, possible to put together headcaps and cervical attachments using plastic belting material which can be cut to size and jointed using a hot knife. This can be done almost as quickly as assembling, adjusting and riveting the ready-made variety, and the finished result is more streamlined and certainly more economic especially if an assistant makes the headgear from measurements, which can be taken very quickly, and the headcap fitted on a subsequent visit.

Attachments can be made to such headgear by punching holes and by melting in hooks of stainless steel. Plastic tubing can be welded to the headgear for the guiding and controlling of curved arms. Cervical straps can be made of such belting and padded with foam strip joined with one of the impact adhesives or self-adhesive Sellotape.

The cervical attachment

A convenient form of cervical attachment is the U-shaped aluminium tube with a foam rubber strip glued to it at the posterior part where pressure is produced on the back of the neck. This tube supports and guides the two extra-oral arms through which traction is brought to the intra-oral appliance, and contains the long elastic band from which the tension is derived (*Figure 7.6*).

The details of the connection between the extra-oral attachment and the upper appliance will vary (*Figure 7.7*).

For the upper appliance that is being used only to retract the upper buccal segments it is most convenient to provide an attachment which plugs into tubes soldered to the first premolar clasps (*Figure 7.7A and B*). This attachment consists of a short labial arch made of 1.0 mm wire and provided with Trevor Johnson friction fit stops (Johnson, 1952) which hold it forwards and well clear of the labial surfaces of the incisors. The extra-oral bow is made from a single piece of heavy wire (1.25 mm) which is wrapped to the smaller arch with soft fine stainless steel wire (0.3 mm) and soldered. The ends of this bow are turned into convenient hooks. Traction is applied to the hooks by looping elastics over them or by forming loops on the ends of the arms that come from the cervical attachment.

Simpler cervical attachments are plastic strips with padding and elastics attached to holes or hooks (*Figure 7.8A–C*).

If the upper appliance is of the kind that is fitted with a free-sliding labial bow for retraction of the

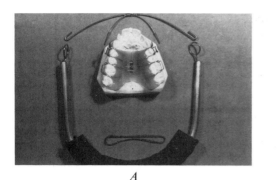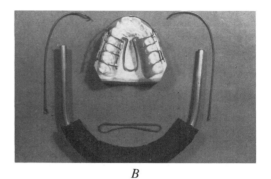

Figure 7.6 Cervical traction appliances using a metal tube and cushion posteriorly; *A*, an extra-oral attachment is plugged into the premolar tubes; *B*, extra-oral arms reach in to engage the free-sliding labial bow

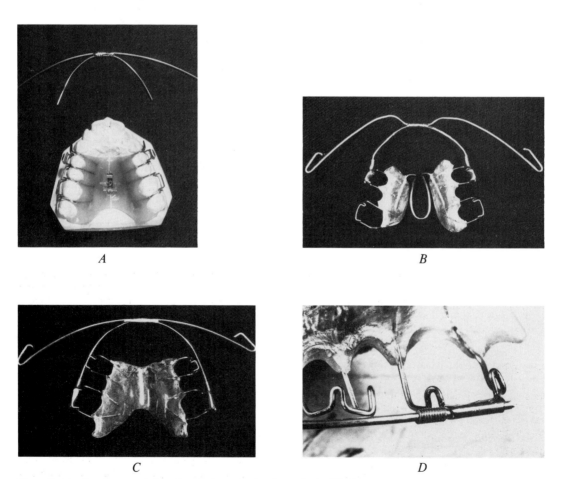

Figure 7.7 *A*, The plug-in arch for tubes on the premolar clasps; *B*, the Kloehn extra-oral attachment; *C*, the standard extra-oral attachment plugged into tubes on the molars; *D*, molar tube soldered to the clasp with a Johnson friction-fit stop on the labial arch

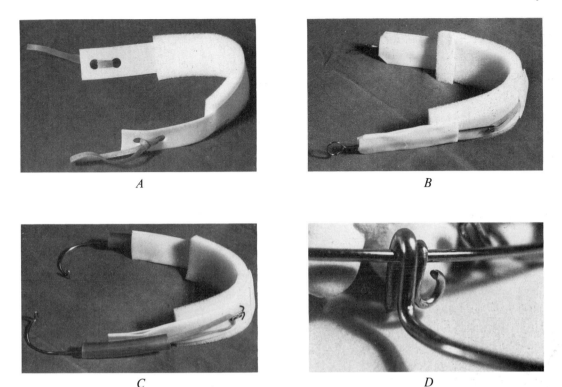

Figure 7.8 Extra-oral headgear; the neckstrap. Neckstraps are made from plastic belting material and are joined by welding with a hot knife or stuck together with double-sided Sellotape; *A*, the simplest neckstrap. The foam padding is fastened with Sellotape and the elastics looped into holes; *B*, traction is conveyed to the 'whiskers' by wires with loops on the ends. The wires run within sleeves of plastic belting at the sides and traction is derived from an elastic in the centre at the back and kept in place by a piece of belting sealed at the edges with a hot knife; *C*, collar with arms running in plastic tubes. Individual elastics are used at either side looped on hooks melted into the plastic; *D*, the ends of the arms are formed into a U and hook onto the free-sliding archwire in front of the stop hook

upper incisors, the arms which emerge from the cervical tube curve forwards and inwards and are formed into hooks which fit over the free-sliding labial arch and impinge on the front of the stop hooks (*Figure 7.8D*).

The headcap

The headcap has the advantage that the direction of pull may be varied in a vertical direction and in some cases it may be thought better to have the pull coming from a higher point than would be possible with cervical traction.

Headcaps are best if of a simple design and consist of a coronal band, an occipital band and a sagittal connector. The lengths of these components are adjusted to determine the height from which the pull is exerted.

A headcap may simply offer a point at which an elastic is hooked or may embody a tube or sleeve which guides and supports an arm which reaches forwards and inwards to hook onto the intra-oral appliance.

The construction of the plastic headcap is shown in *Figures 7.9* and *7.10*. Should there be any reason why plastic material cannot be used, the headcap can be made of webbing and sewn together as was formerly the normal practice.

There are three methods of attaching elastics to the plastic headcap; holes may be punched, through which different lengths of elastics may be looped at different points to adjust the strength of the pull; hooks may be placed by heating the metal and welding them into the plastic; tubes may be welded on in which arms run and the elastic attached to holes, hooks or by slitting the end of the tube and jamming the elastic in the slit.

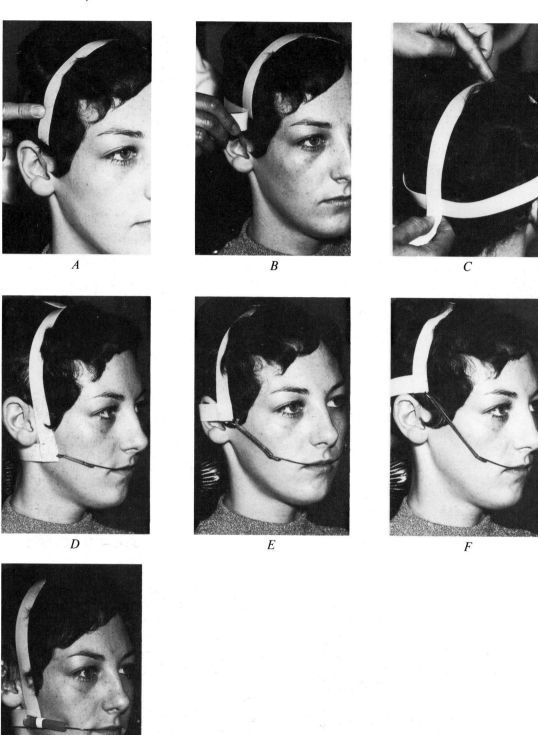

Figure 7.9 Construction of the headcap. *A–C*, measuring the tape; *D–F*, low, medium and high-pull headcaps; *G*, headcap with tube to guide the arm which reaches into the intra-oral appliance

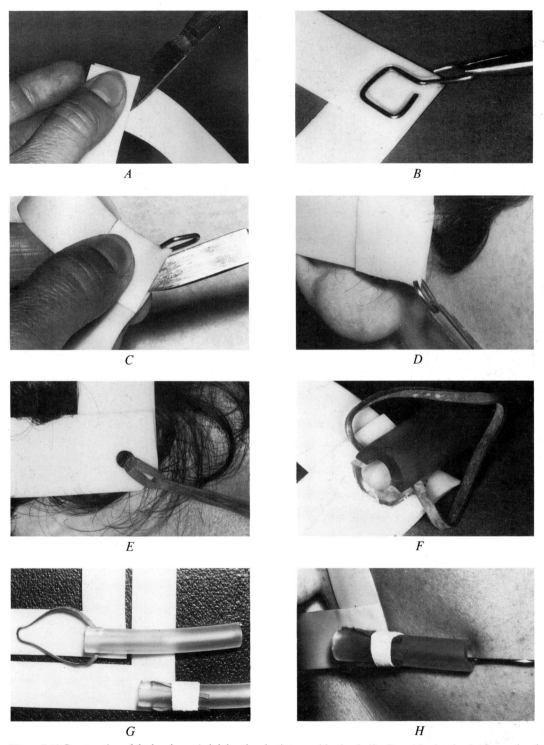

Figure 7.10 Construction of the headcap; *A*, joining the plastic tape with a hot knife; *B*, melting in a hook; *C*, securing the hook with a patch of tape; *D*, the hook used for attachment of elastic; *E*, attachment of elastic through a hole punched in the tape; *F* and *G*, fixing elastic in a guide tube, the end of the elastic turned back, taped down with adhesive plaster; *H*, the guide tube with extra-oral arm in use

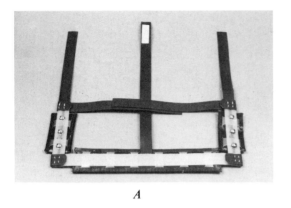

A

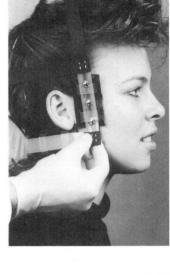

B

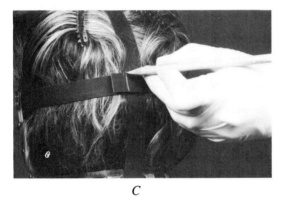

C

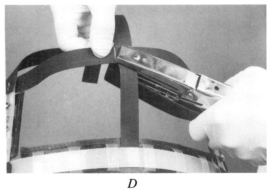

D

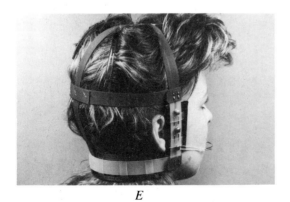

E

Figure 7.11 *A*, Headcap prior to stapling; *B*, selection of the correct size; *C*, after stapling the sagittal and coronal bands the occipital band is marked with a wax pencil; *D*, stapling the occipital band with a heavy-duty stapler. The ends of the staples are flattened with Universal Pliers; *E*, final position of the stapled bands; *F*, elastic force applied along the occlusal plane by the lowermost hook

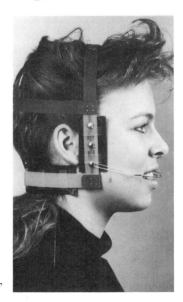

F

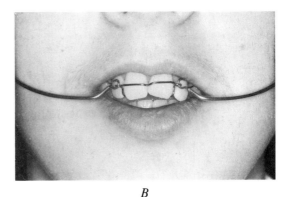

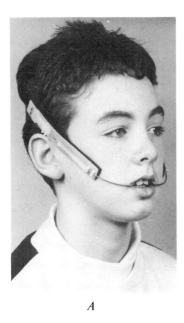

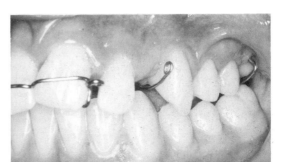

Figure 7.12 *A*, 'J' hook headgear; *B* and *C*, attachment of the 'J' hooks to an intra-oral bow of 0.7 mm wire by means of loops in the bow.

Ready-made headgear, available from many suppliers of orthodontic materials, may be preferred to the tailor-made headcap on the grounds of speed and convenience. Ready-made headcaps incorporate adjustments to suit different head sizes and permit variation in the direction and amount of tension that can be applied to the orthodontic appliance. An example is shown in *Figure 7.11* and this is one of many that are available from a number of manufacturers.

Extra-oral traction can be usefully employed in a number of other situations as, for instance, where reinforcement of intra-oral anchorage may be required. Such a need may arise, for example, where intra-oral appliances are being used for the retroclination of upper incisors and there is a risk of anchorage slippage. Another good example is where lingual root torque is being applied to the upper incisors as here there is a considerable forward reaction exerted on the teeth in the buccal segments.

Such anchorage may be attached to an appliance through 'whiskers', also available ready-made, and plugged into molar or premolar tubes, as previously described, and using a force just enough to stabilize anchorage. 'J' hook headgear may be applied to a labial bow constructed from 0.7 mm wire with coils formed to receive the hooks (*Figure 7.12*). An upwards direction of pull improves the retention of the appliance and may be easier for the patient to wear when anchorage for distal movement of buccal teeth is required.

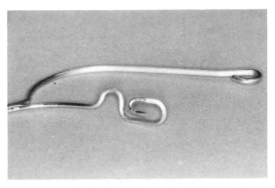

Figure 7.13 Safety facebow. The ends of the intra-oral part of the bow are recurved so presenting a smooth loop to lie against the soft tissues of the lips and cheeks.

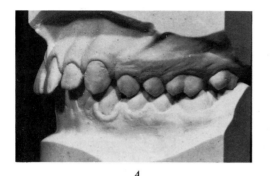

A

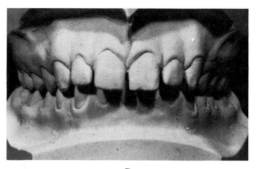

B

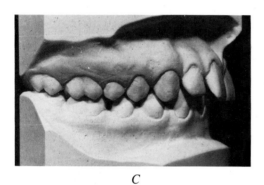

C

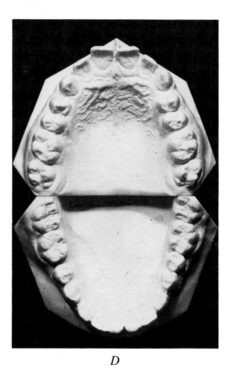

D

Figure 7.14 Treatment of unilateral postnormal occlusion with unilateral intermaxillary traction. Patient has excellent arch form and dental base relation with spacing in upper and lower arch but was self-conscious about the upper incisor spacing and slight prominence; *A–D*, before treatment; *E–H*, appearance five years after correction of the unilateral malocclusion (five years after treatment); *I* and *J*, full face and profile (five years after treatment)

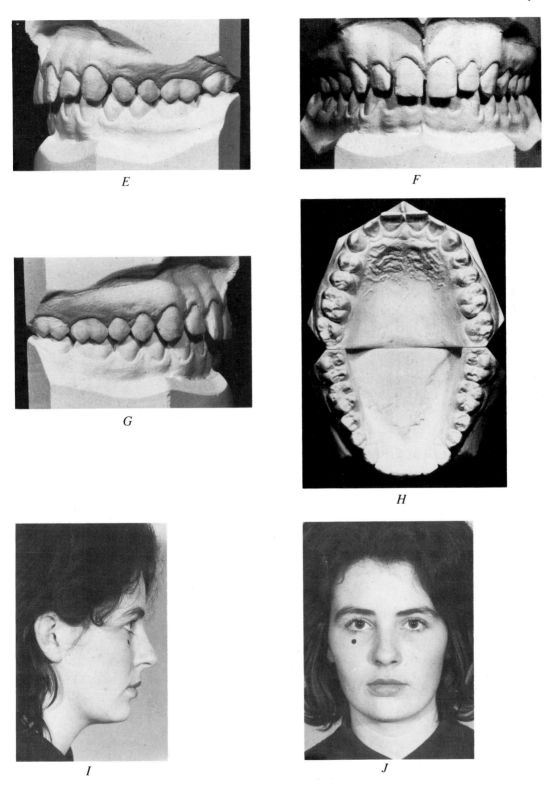

Figure 7.14 continued

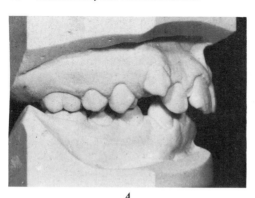

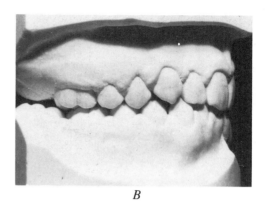

A   B

Figure 7.15 Patient with prominence of upper anterior teeth and scissors bite on the right premolars. Treated with extra-oral traction and correction of scissors bite on the right side; *A*, before treatment; *B*, after treatment

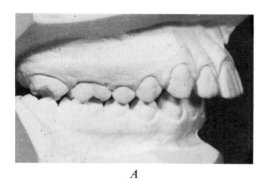

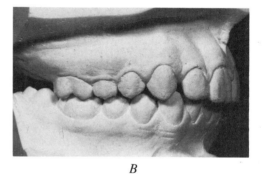

A   B

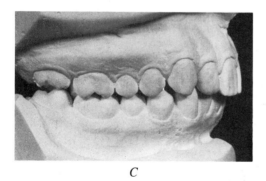

C

Figure 7.16 Classical Class II division 1 malocclusion. There was no spacing in the lower arch and it was decided to treat by extraction of upper second molars and extra-oral traction; *A*, before treatment; *B*, second molars have been removed and the arch discrepancy corrected by extra-oral traction to the upper arch; *C*, upper third molars have erupted and the occlusion has stabilized although there was a very slight relapse

When using headgear it is important to ensure that the ends of all extra-oral parts are smooth and that clear instructions are given for using and wearing the appliance so as to avoid accidental injury to the patient. Safety headgears are available which disassemble if a sudden increase of pressure should occur. A safety facebow (*Figure 7.13*), has a recurved intra-oral end which reduces the risk of injury should it become accidentally dislodged.

Extra-oral traction may also be applied to the lower arch in Class III malocclusion. The principles are the same; a baseplate is fitted and means found of extending the baseplate outside the mouth using a 'whisker' type of extra-oral attachment or by bringing the arms of the extra-oral traction apparatus inside the mouth and hooking it onto the appliance at some convenient spot.

Figures 7.14–7.17 show a group of subjects in which intermaxillary and extra-oral traction were used in treatment.

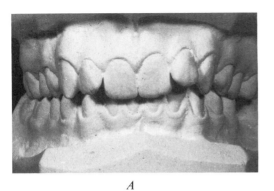

A

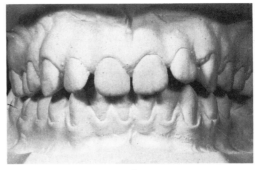

C

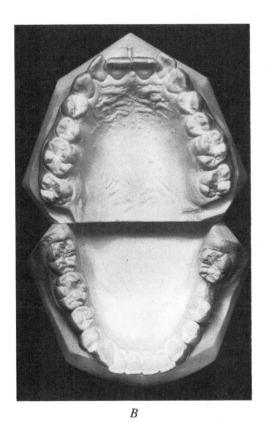

B

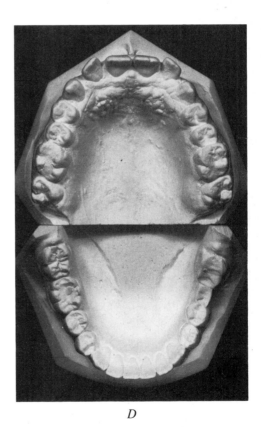

D

Figure 7.17 Records of a patient aged 16 years with slight Class II division 2 malocclusion and absence of third molars. There were many restorations including the need for a bridge for the left lower first molar. Lower arch form was excellent. A conservative approach was decided on by extra-oral traction with an upper removable appliance; *A* and *B*, before treatment; *C* and *D*, buccal segments have been moved distally and spacing has developed in the upper incisor region; *E* and *F*, the lateral incisors have been over-rotated mesiolingually. This position was maintained for 9 months with a removable appliance; *G* and *H*, three years out of retention. Some lower arch restorations are being completed

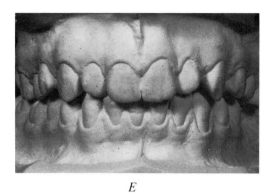

E

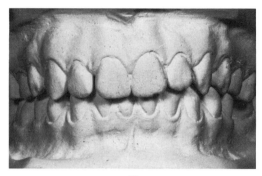

G

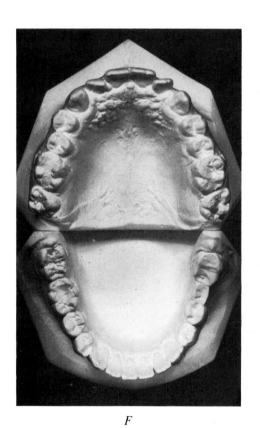

F

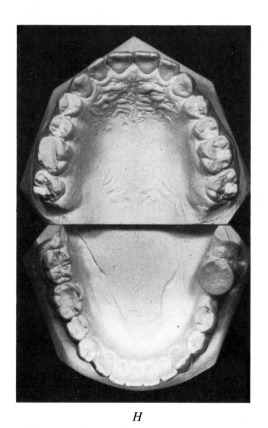

H

Figure 7.17 continued

Chapter 8

Functional appliances

Like the man who discovered that he had been speaking prose for years without realizing it, it is possible that orthodontists have for long been using functional appliances without thinking of the appliances in question as functional. Biting planes, whether flat or inclined, and the oral screen are functional appliances and the many, more complex, systems available today are extensions, elaborations and combinations of the two aspects of orofacial function employed in the 'plane' and the 'screen' type of appliance. Further activities introduced by the inclusion of elastic, pressure-storing elements into the appliances add a further dimension to the mechanical complexities.

Functional appliances act either through the media of the masticatory muscles, which have both their origins and insertions in bone, or through the craniofacial and lingual muscles, which have their origins or insertions or both in soft tissues.

Functional appliances can be either placed between and against the teeth, concentrating the pressures of the musculature on individual teeth or groups of teeth, or placed about the teeth, screening them from the pressures of the tongue, lips and cheeks.

Functional appliances may also combine these effects and by their presence in the mouth must inevitably do so to a greater or lesser degree.

Another effect of functional appliances is to modify the pattern of movement of the mandible. This effect must occur coincidentally with many functional appliances and while the plan may be to devise means of influencing the positions of teeth, effects may also be produced on the mandible by accident. If the widest context is envisaged, then it is conceivable that effects may be produced on the face as a whole.

It is, indeed, such a concept that seems to inspire some of the more sanguine philosophies of function-al appliance methodology in urging that appropriate functional therapy will engender facial development of a degree that can compensate for the all too obvious defects of nature in individual cases.

There is a parallel with the belief of Edward Angle that if the teeth were mechanically placed in correct relationships by fixed appliance therapy there would be a development of the facial structures to correspond with the new dental alignment (Angle, 1907, 1910).

It would sometimes appear to be the belief of functional therapists that the same fortunate outcome is achievable by using the influence of function, which is one of the more important reasons for the existence of the organism, and that function is a more natural influence than mechanical treatment and thereby likely to be more effective.

The possible connections between functional appliance therapy and facial growth in general will be discussed in due course.

Simple functional appliances

The bite-plane and the oral screen illustrate in their simplest forms the principles of functional appliances operating through, firstly, the muscles of mastication and, secondly, the musculature of the face and tongue.

Bite-planes

Bite-planes may be divided into planes which lie parallel to the occlusal plane and planes inclined at an angle to the occlusal plane.

Bite-planes lying parallel to the occlusal plane (sometimes called horizontal bite-planes) are designed to produce mainly axial stresses on the teeth. Such planes are intended either to prop the bite temporarily to facilitate certain tooth movements or to cause certain adjustments of the vertical relationships of the teeth.

Inclined bite-planes are designed to produce stresses lateral to the axes of the teeth and thereby lead to their movement in a lateral direction.

The anterior bite-plane

This consists of a platform behind the upper incisor teeth on which the lower incisors bite (*Figure 8.1*).

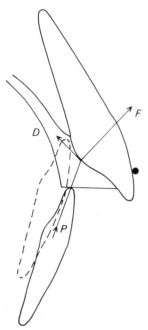

Figure 8.1 The anterior bite-plane. Overbite is increased (dotted lines) and the anterior bite-plane is placed and the lower incisors bite upon it. The upper incisors are restrained by a labial bow. The pressure of the bite, *P*, acting on the sloping surface of the upper incisors produces a forward component, *F*, which tends to procline the upper teeth and a distal and upward component, *D*, parallel to the slope on the tooth. If the bite-plane sinks, the labial bow moves forward with it and cannot restrain the upper incisors

Formerly, the plane was simple in construction and was often used with a labial bow of heavy wire. The reason for the labial bow has nowhere been explained, but it would seem that as the pressure of the bite falls on the plane, the slopes of the cingula of the upper anterior teeth would produce an anterior component of force and so cause proclination of these teeth and a sinking of the baseplate into the gum tissues behind the upper incisors. The labial bow was intended to prevent these unwanted effects occurring, but the arrangement is not altogether effective.

The purpose of the anterior bite-plane usually is to reduce the overbite of the anterior teeth. It was formerly thought that the overbite reduction was brought about by depressing the lower anterior teeth into the alveolar bone but this is now known not to occur and that, on the contrary, the lower incisors continue to erupt in many cases.

Investigation has shown that when the bite is propped on an upper anterior bite-plane, far from the anterior teeth becoming depressed, the posterior teeth, relieved of the pressure of mastication, erupt further and when the bite-plane is removed, it is found that the overbite of the anterior teeth is reduced (Richardson and Adams, 1963). This effect is known as 'opening the bite' and must be distinguished from a purely temporary propping of the bite for the purpose of facilitating tooth movement, such as moving an anterior tooth across the bite of the lower teeth.

The effect of the pressure of an anterior bite-plane falling on the sloping lingual surfaces of the upper anterior teeth, thereby proclining them, has long been recognized and various solutions devised, one of which was the labial bow mentioned above.

Sved (1944) introduced a bite-plane which covered the incisal edges of the upper anterior teeth thereby ensuring that the pressure of the bite was transmitted axially to the teeth and eliminating the forward component of force tending to their proclination (*Figure 8.2*).

The Sved bite-plane is the most satisfactory answer to the problem of supporting the bite while the posterior teeth are allowed to erupt and thereby to open the bite or reduce the anterior overbite. It is necessary, however, to ensure that oral hygiene is scrupulously maintained and the appliance must be worn at all times and in particular at mealtimes. It is necessary that the patient adapts to eating with the appliance in place and cuts up food so that this can be done as easily as possible. The plate and mouth must be meticulously cleaned after meals and the patient must not eat sweets.

The question has to be considered as to what happens after an anterior bite-plane, as just described, is removed. It has been noted that the effect of such a plane is to increase the height of the face by permitting the posterior teeth to erupt and if the appliance is then removed, the pressure of the occlusion will fall on the back teeth once again.

In theory, the position of the mandible is an element or link in the muscular chain made up of the post-cervical musculature, through the epicranial aponeurosis and its musculature, the facial and masticatory musculature and the precervical system, linking all anteriorly to the thorax and sternum. Moreover, theory has it that face height is only one dimension in this chain and that the development of the dentition takes place within the constraints of

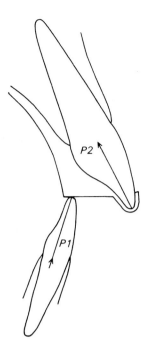

Figure 8.2 A Sved bite-plane caps the upper incisors and the bite pressure *P1* is transmitted axially, *P2*, to the upper incisors. Any forward component is resisted because the Sved plate prevents tipping labially of the upper incisors. After a period of wear, eruption of the back teeth will result in a reduction of overbite when the appliance is removed

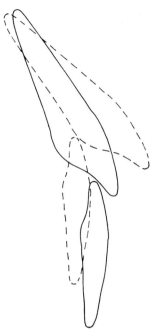

Figure 8.3 After the overbite has been reduced, the upper incisors may be retroclined, space conditions permitting, and the new incisor relation, in the presence of normal soft tissue posture and function, remains stable

the face height so imposed, and that dental development cannot actually influence face height. This would mean that an increase in face height produced by causing eruption of back teeth must return to its original dimension after appliances used to produce the change are withdrawn.

In practice there seems to be greater flexibility in the human organism than is implied by these ideas. Experience shows that anterior overbites reduced by the use of anterior bite-planes may remain reduced after appliances are withdrawn, and in others they may not. It is, therefore, important not to use such a bite-plane without a plan as to what is to be done when overbite has been reduced (*Figure 8.3*).

It would seem that in young patients, having a full complement of teeth and growing actively, considerable changes are taking place in the shape and size of the face as a whole and modifications induced in the pattern of the dentition by functional appliances, such as bite-planes, can become incorporated in occlusal morphology as permanent features.

On the other hand, when growth slows down and ceases, modifications of the face and occlusion are less easily produced by means of bite-planes and less easily maintained when appliances are withdrawn.

Figure 8.4 shows the casts of a patient aged 14 years who was referred because of a close bite of the Angle Class II division 2 type with trauma to the lingual gingival margin of the upper incisors. The patient was given a Sved bite-plane for 4 months by which time the overbite of the incisor teeth had markedly diminished. The appliance was worn for a further 9 months at night-time only and then discarded. The new overbite relationship remained stable.

The uses of anterior bite-planes

The most frequent use of the anterior bite-plane is to reduce the overbite of the anterior teeth as a preliminary to the reduction of overjet associated with proclination of the upper anterior teeth. In these circumstances, the lower incisors may be biting on the lingual surfaces of the upper anterior teeth at points towards the cingula of these teeth or at the gum margins of the upper teeth or at points on the palatal mucosa some distance behind the gum margins. It is clearly necessary to reduce the overbite before retroclining the proclined upper anterior teeth. The Sved bite-plane will do this.

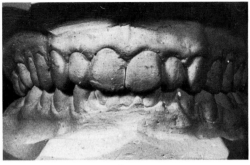
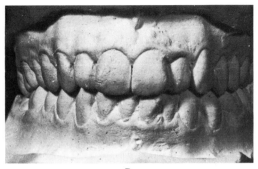

A   *B*

Figure 8.4 Reduction of incisor overbite relationship. The overbite relationship of the incisors is a complex of interincisal angle, dental base relationship, face height, soft-tissue posture and function. The patient in this record had a favourable tooth environment apart from interincisal angle. As the lower incisors were traumatizing the upper lingual gum margin, *A*, the patient was given a Sved anterior bite-plane and the overbite reduced and remained stable without any further treatment, *B*

There must also be space in the upper dental arch to make the distal and lingual movements of the upper anterior teeth possible (*Figure 8.3*).

It may be that the upper anterior teeth are already spaced as well as proclined, but if not, then space must be created by extraction of teeth at appropriate points. Extraction of first premolars provides space at a convenient place in the arch but extraction of other teeth may be more appropriate.

In correcting proclination of upper incisors, the incisors are retroclined but canine, premolar and molar teeth are moved mesiodistally to make available the necessary space.

Important points in the eventual stability of overbite reduction and correction of incisor relationship are the interincisal angle and the resting posture and function of the tongue and lips. If the interincisal angle and degree of overbite are average, and lip and tongue posture and function are normal, the conditions for stability are present. Excessive interincisal angle and anomalies of lip and tongue posture and function militate against a permanent result.

Other uses of anterior bite-planes

The treatment of pain associated with the temporomandibular joint sometimes entails the use of bite-planes designed to free existing occlusal contacts which often are abnormal due to loss of teeth and tilting of the remaining teeth and the presence of high spots in the occlusal planes. Often there is an increased incisor overbite of considerable degree. It is common practice to fit a thin overlay over all the teeth in one dental arch in order to eliminate abnormal and premature contacts on closure and so to mitigate the possible effects of clenching the teeth, whether during the daytime or at night.

One possible drawback of an overlay over the back teeth can be that depression of these teeth may take place thus worsening any tendency there may be to increased incisor overbite.

In these circumstances, the use of an anterior bite-plane of the Sved type has advantages in that premature and abnormal contacts are eliminated and any effect on occlusal levels in the dental arches can only be of a beneficial nature tending, as such an appliance may do, to reduce incisor overbite.

The lower inclined plane

The lower inclined plane is an appliance used for the treatment of an incorrect biting relationship of the upper and lower incisors, when one or a number of upper incisors bite lingually to the lower incisors. The appliance consists of a polished metal or acrylic resin plane inclined at about 45° to the occlusal plane and placed between the upper and lower incisors in such a way that the upper incisor or incisors bite on the plane and are guided into their correct positions labially to the lower incisors (*Figure 8.5*).

Indications and contraindications for the use of the lower inclined plane

The lower inclined plane is useful when the incisor teeth are at a relatively early stage of eruption and where there is a good degree of overbite. In cases where many deciduous teeth have been removed, rendering the temporary propping open of the bite difficult, the inclined plane is useful.

If there is a marked degree of mandibular prognathism and the overbite of the incisors is not great the inclined plane should not be used. It may be impossible to produce the necessary degree of

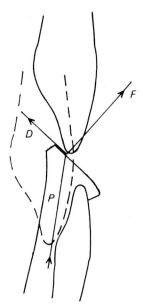

Figure 8.5 The lower inclined plane caps the lower incisors and is inclined at about 45° to the occlusal plane. On closing, the upper incisors which formerly bit behind the lower incisors now bite on the plane and the pressure of the bite, *P*, develops a component at right angles to the plane, *F*, and a component along the plane, *D*. The pressure *F* proclines the upper incisors. If there is any element of forward displacement of the mandible, the amount of movement of the upper incisors needed may be quite small

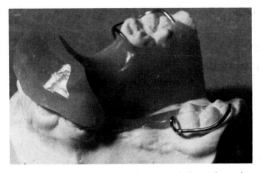

Figure 8.6 A lower removable inclined plane clasped on the lower first permanent molars. If there are no back teeth the buccal gum pads should be covered with extensions of the baseplate

upper incisor proclination and if the overbite becomes reduced it may be impossible to produce correct incisor relationship in the end.

Design and construction of the lower inclined plane

The most satisfactory inclined plane is the removable, clear acrylic plane. Sometimes cemented inclined planes and planes in cast metal such as silver are recommended, but both have drawbacks. If a plane is cemented, it is impossible to check progress in the tooth movement unless the appliance is removed, and this may entail damaging the plane. Cast metal planes are not worth the time and expense of construction because removable acrylic planes are equally effective and much less troublesome to construct and for the patient to wear.

A removable acrylic plane is made on a stone model from an alginate impression.

Clasps should be used if there are suitable teeth present (*Figure 8.6*). If all the lower back teeth have been removed, as occasionally happens, the baseplate should be thickened a little and carried over the occlusal surface of the gum pads. The resulting flanges help the patient in retaining the appliance.

The inclined plane is built up, capping the incisor and canine teeth, and the appliance is made in clear acrylic material.

When fitting the appliance, any undercuts in the resin due to tilted or imbricated teeth should be removed until the appliance goes in easily.

The inclined plane is adjusted for height and angulation by grinding the slope against a 3 inch rotating lathe wheel. The plane is finally polished.

The appliance should be worn full-time and the patient instructed to cut up food and adopt a soft diet until the incisor relationship is correct and the appliance can be removed (*Figure 8.7*).

Treatment should only take a matter of weeks and if improvement does not appear to be taking place soon, a check should be made on the wearing of the appliance and the diagnosis of the case.

The oral screen

The oral screen is a functional appliance by virtue of the fact that it embodies no active elements designed to produce forces acting on the teeth but produces its effects by redirecting the pressures of the muscular and soft-tissue curtain of the cheeks and lips.

The oral screen is also used at times to counteract deficiencies in lip posture and function by providing a covering for the anterior teeth and their adjoining gingival tissues and to prevent oral respiration when anterior and posterior oral seals are inadequate.

The value of the oral screen in producing improvements in tooth arrangement and occlusal relationship, in training the labial musculature to improvement in posture and function, in improving the health of the pharyngeal tissues by preventing oral respiration, and through all these means promoting the greater well-being of the patient, has long been a matter of debate. The evidence for the more remote effects and wider implications of

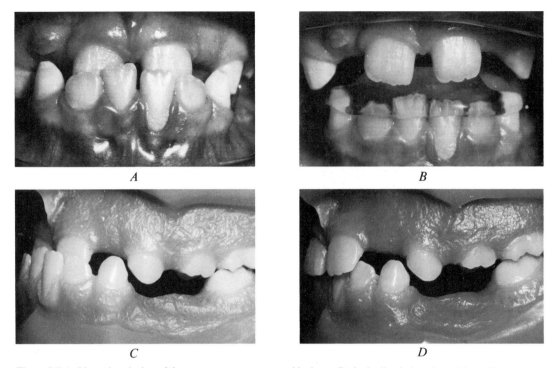

Figure 8.7 *A*, Lingual occlusion of the upper permanent central incisors; *B*, the inclined plane in position with upper incisors biting on it; *C* and *D*, photographs of acrylic models of the patient shown in *A* and *B*; *C*, before treatment, *D*, after treatment

treatment with the oral screen has been largely subjective, difficult to record precisely and to distinguish among the changes which could be attributed to growth, development and variations in the health of patients treated with this appliance.

It is in the region of the lips and labial segments of the dental arches that the oral screen can be used to produce predictable treatment results, and here the effects which the oral screen produces can be recorded with some accuracy and objectivity.

If the upper incisors are proclined and spaced and there is an increase in overjet and the oral screen is made so that it touches only the proclined incisors and is not in contact with the teeth in the buccal segments, the pressure of the lips and of the cheeks which lie in contact with the smooth divergent lateral wings of the oral screen will all be concentrated on the labial surfaces of the proclined incisors near the incisal edges (*Figures 8.8* and *8.9A*). If the lower incisors are in contact with the upper incisors in the position of centric occlusion, pressure of the oral screen will be transmitted also to the lower incisors when the teeth are brought together as in swallowing, and this contact of the upper incisors with the lowers will prevent retroclination of the upper incisors (*Figure 8.9B*).

The use of an oral screen in circumstances such as

these is not without risk to the upper incisor teeth, which are pressed from in front by the oral screen and intermittently tapped from behind by the lower incisors at each closure of the teeth into occlusion. In the course of time resorption of the upper root apices may occur.

If, when the posterior teeth are in occlusion, there is no contact between the upper and lower incisors, there will be no obstacle to a lingual movement of the upper incisors (*Figure 8.9A*) and the upper incisors may be retroclined by means of the oral screen.

In designing an oral screen the relationship of the lower lip to the labial segments of the dental arches is important. In cases in which there is such a degree of overjet that it is only with difficulty that the lower lip can be brought out over the upper incisors, care must be taken to curve the oral screen inwards towards the lower incisors sufficiently to allow the lower lip to slide easily upwards and outwards labially to the oral screen. If, in these circumstances, the screen is brought downwards in a continuous curve over the upper incisors the lower lip may not succeed in reaching out in front of the screen and, lying inside it, may force the screen out of position and expel it from the mouth, or else, reaching out in front of the screen, it may exert such pressure on its labial surface as to rock the upper edge forwards out of control of the upper lip. In either event, the screen cannot be tolerated by the patient.

The mechanical action of the oral screen can be seen, therefore, to be in producing a lingual pressure on the upper incisors, and lingual inclination of these teeth if there is no mechanical obstacle to such a movement. The possibility of producing more far-reaching alterations in occlusal relationship, such as reduction in overbite and correction of postnormality of the occlusion, has been suggested from time to time, but the authors have not found the oral screen to be effective in these respects.

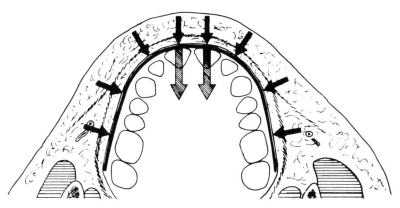

Figure 8.8 The oral screen. The entire pressure of the soft tissues of the lips and cheeks is concentrated on the central incisors. The lateral pressure of the cheeks on the smooth sloping surface of the screen is resolved in a posterior direction. The appliance may be designed to act upon the lateral incisors as well

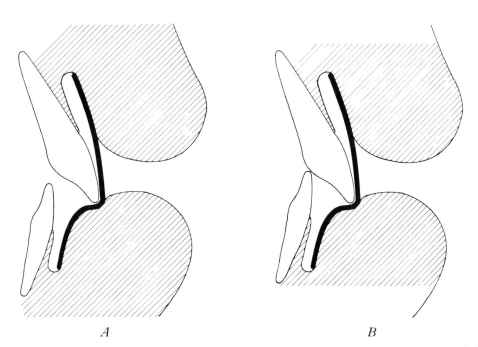

A   *B*

Figure 8.9 *A*, An oral screen fitted in a case in which the upper incisors are proclined and spaced but the lower incisors do not touch the upper incisors when the teeth are in centric occlusion. In these circumstances the oral screen will retrocline the upper incisors; *B*, an oral screen fitted in a case in which there is proclination of the upper incisors and the lower incisors touch the upper incisors when the teeth are in centric occlusion. In this situation, the pressure of the oral screen on the upper incisors is transmitted to the lower incisors. It is doubtful whether the upper incisors can be retroclined by the use of an oral screen in a case like this

Construction of the oral screen

The oral screen is constructed on upper and lower working models fixed together in centric occlusion. The impressions from which the models are cast must reproduce the full depth of the labial sulcus.

One thickness of pink wax is applied to the labial aspect of the teeth and the alveolar processes and extended to the limits of the sulcus vertically and distally, allowance being made for the labial and buccal fraena by trimming the wax as required. This layer of wax is sealed in position and then scraped down over the incisal third of the labial surfaces of the upper incisor teeth which it is desired to retrocline (*Figure 8.10*). The thickness of modelling

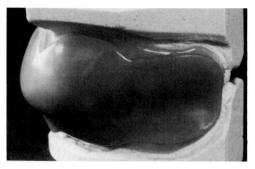

Figure 8.11 The oral screen waxed up on the models

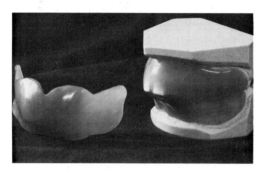

Figure 8.10 The models are fixed in centric occlusion with plaster or wax and covered on the labial aspect with a layer of wax. Note how the wax curves inwards below the upper incisors. The waxed oral screen is on the left

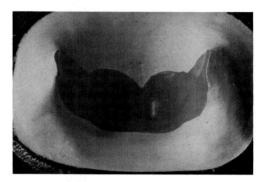

Figure 8.12 The oral screen encased in the lower half of the flask before pouring the top half

wax is not standardized and if the wax used is not thick enough, additions must be made to the sides of the wax layer in order to leave sufficient clearance between the oral screen and the teeth and alveolar tissues in the buccal region.

Attention must also be paid to the contour of the wax between the incisal edges of the upper incisor and the lower labial sulcus to ensure that the correct curve is provided to accept the lower lip.

The oral screen is then constructed in a single thickness of wax over the surface provided on the working models. The edges of the wax model of the oral screen are made a little less than the limits of the buccal vestibule and allowance is made for the labial and buccal fraena (*Figure 8.11*). The wax of the oral screen can be thickened as may seem necessary to make the final appliance strong enough.

The screen is then chilled and invested, outer aspect downwards, in a thin cold plaster mix. As a precaution against warpage during investment, the screen, while still on the model, may be coated with a layer of plaster. When the plaster has set, the coated screen is removed and invested in the deep part of the flask (*Figure 8.12*). The second half of the flask is poured into the inside of the screen. The

appliance is finished in clear acrylic resin and smoothed and polished.

If the oral screen is being used to retrocline the upper incisor teeth, additions of clear, cold-curing acrylic material may be made to the inside of the appliance as tooth movement takes place, to maintain pressure on the anterior teeth.

The effect of the oral screen in retroclining the upper incisors is shown in *Figure 8.13*.

Functional jaw orthopaedics

Functional jaw orthopaedics is the system of orthodontic treatment which makes use of forces which act in and about the human dentition during the activities of the masticatory face. In suitable cases, treatment with functional appliances offers a means of treating severe malocclusions simply, but it should also be borne in mind that such treatment applied to conditions for which it is not suited can be ineffectual.

Functional jaw orthopaedics embraces treatment with any of the appliances in which loose-fitting devices are placed between or about the teeth, so redirecting the pressures of the facial or masticatory

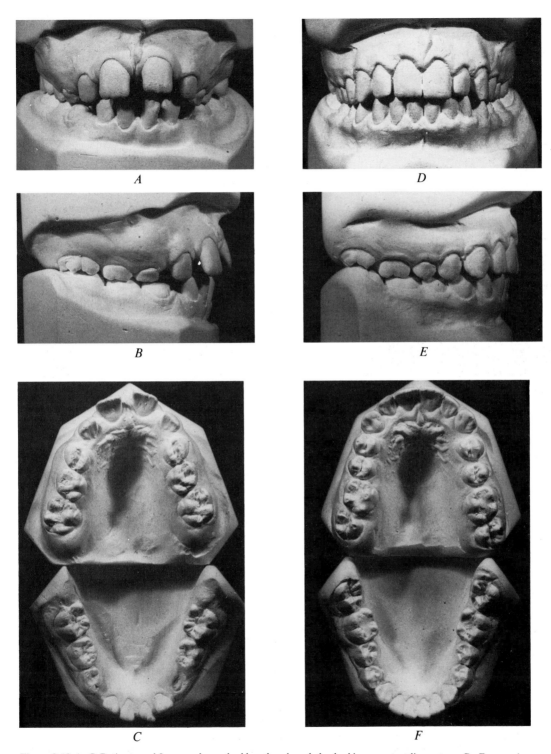

Figure 8.13 *A–C*, Patient aged 8 years who sucked her thumb and also had incompetent lip posture; *D–F*, an oral screen was used and at age 12 the condition had completely resolved. It is probable that the oral screen acted as a substitute for the thumb habit and that soft tissue patterning matured over the ensuing years. From records kindly lent by Professor A. Richardson

muscles on to the teeth and their supporting structures in such ways as to produce improvements in tooth arrangements and occlusal relations.

The most well-known systematic approach to the design and use of functional appliances was that of Andresen (1936), although Robin (1902) anticipated the general shape of the appliance or 'monobloc' that is used in the Andresen system. Whatever the name of the appliance that is used, the purpose is to produce a redirection of the forces of mastication that are already at play within and about the oral cavity until such time as premeditated changes in tooth arrangement and occlusal relationship have been brought about.

While the functional appliances of Andresen redirect the pressures produced by the muscles of mastication on the teeth, the approach of Fränkel (1966) is different in that Fränkel's method is one in which the pressures of the tongue, lips and cheeks are prevented from impinging upon the teeth and alveolar processes by means of a 'Function Corrector' or 'Function Regulator', and so produce changes in the growth patterns of these structures.

Theoretical principles

The foundation on which functional orthopaedics of the jaws rests is the theory of 'functional adaptation' evolved by Roux (1895) conceived as a principle which determines the arrangement of the teeth and the form of the jaws in which the dentition is placed. Haupl *et al.* (1952) have embodied the conception of the treatment of malocclusion by functional means in the following quotation from their textbook:

Tissue-forming functional stimuli originate from the activity of the tongue, lip, facial and masticatory muscles. These stimuli are transmitted to the teeth, paradontal tissue, alveolar bone and mandibular joint through a passive, loose-fitting appliance inserted between the teeth, the result being that the transmitted stimuli induce the desired changes in the tissues affected.

The theoretical basis of the system of functional treatment suggests that the new pattern of function dictated by the appliance or activator leads to the development of a correspondingly new morphological pattern, not only of tooth arrangement and occlusion, but also of facial size and proportions. If this is so, then it should be possible from the study of treated cases to show at what sites and to what degree changes in form have taken place within the jaws, temporomandibular joints and dentoalveolar structures.

Today it is acknowledged that dramatic and permanent improvements in occlusal relationships can be produced by functional appliances in some cases. The changes in the occlusion can be seen and estimated clinically with considerable accuracy by means of the teeth, which do not alter in size and shape, but the nature and extent of the accompanying changes in the shape of the jaws and face are less easy to measure, especially as growth in these areas may have taken place at the same time as the treatment procedures were carried out.

It is believed by many advocates of functional jaw orthopaedics, on the basis of clinical experience, that changes occur at the condyle of the mandible as a result of stimulation of growth at this site leading to increase in mandibular length. Korkhaus (1960), from the cephalometric examination of Class II division 1 malocclusion treated by activators, suggested that the changes in mandibular conformation rapidly produced correction of the occlusal relationship, and hence no changes in tooth position within the jaws were necessary; not only did this make for a more stable end result, but also there was no risk to the periodontal tissues as a result of the orthodontic treatment.

An investigation into the effects produced by functional appliances in the treatment of Class II division 1 malocclusion had previously been carried out by Softley (1953) with the aid of cephalometric X-ray analysis. This author found that while after treatment with activator appliances considerable changes had taken place in tooth inclination, particularly upper incisor inclination and in alveolar prognathism, changes in basal prognathism, other than changes attributable to growth, could not be detected.

Moss (1962) analysed the results of activator treatment of 30 cases of Class II division 1 malocclusion. Using cephalometric X-ray films, Moss found that in 76% of cases there was a forward growth difference of the lower jaw in relation to the upper, the lower jaw growing forwards more rapidly than the upper by 1 mm per year. Moss explained this result in terms of a releasing of inhibiting factors in the growth of the lower jaw through the use of the activator.

Björk (1963) in a personal communication has shown by the cephalometric X-ray study of growth and development in Class II division 1 cases that while the dental base relationship may remain unchanged as growth proceeds, this relationship may in some cases improve towards normality and in others deteriorate to a more severe degree of postnormality. Such growth changes as these modify to a great degree the response of cases of postnormal occlusion when treatment is carried out by activators. Favourable growth changes, taking place during treatment, accelerate the improvements in occlusal relationship brought about by functional appliances. In contrast, the absence of favourable growth changes or the deterioration in dental base relationship will delay or prevent entirely any correction of occlusal relationship by means of activator treatment.

Björk, in a personal communication, has stated that:

Treatment is divided into three types according to the growth trend of the sagittal jaw relationship.

1. If the sagittal jaw relationship is postnormal but is growing towards normality, that is to say, if lower prognathism is increasing in relation to upper prognathism, then prognosis is good. In such circumstances, an activator or even a bite-plate will be sufficient to produce the required result. The appliance will function by growth adaptation in that it removes distal intercuspidation and thereby makes it possible for the occlusion to develop in the normal direction in the same degree as the sagittal jaw relation. Occipital traction on the upper molars will have the same effect during growth adaptation in that the distal intercuspidation is removed. Tooth movement of other kinds is not required. In cases with normal spacing, extraction is not necessary and the treatment should be done before the end of puberal growth.

2. Where prognathism is developing at the same rate in both jaws, the jaw relationship remains unchanged. Here it is necessary to treat the malocclusion by means of tooth movement. Fixed appliances are most useful in combination with occipital traction. In such cases, occipital traction moves the teeth, and tooth movement may be easier if certain teeth are extracted in one or both jaws. Removable appliances such as the activator can be used with good prospects where there is considerable growth in alveolar height, but in these cases treatment must then be done before the end of puberal growth.

3. If prognathism of the upper jaw is increasing in relation to the lower, treatment is difficult. Removable appliances are contraindicated if they remove the intercuspidation which is the natural compensatory occlusal mechanism. Treatment has to be done by tooth movement with fixed appliances in combination with occipital traction and extraction in both jaws. Tooth movement has to compensate for increased deterioration in the sagittal jaw relation. For this reason, treatment may be done late, after pubertal growth, and the finished treatment has to be retained with occlusal stabilization.

It is clear that while the decision to carry out orthodontic treatment by means of functional appliances must rest to a great extent upon a multitude of clinical observations and assessments, the effects of treatment cannot be explained by anything less than the most precise measuring methods available, and much remains to be discovered about the details of the effects produced by functional appliances.

Further theoretical advantages arising from the use of functional appliances concern the reaction of the periodontal tissues to the influence of activators in pressing on the teeth. The pressure exerted by activators differs from the pressure exerted by active appliances, or appliances embodying sources of stored pressure, in that activator pressure is intermittent even while the appliance is being worn, and also this intermittent pressure is only applied for a proportion of the 24 hours, as activators are usually only worn at night. The pressure exerted by active appliances is continuous, the appliances being worn all of the 24 hours. The effect of activators is to impose impulses or shocks to the teeth and their surrounding structures, such impulses being under the control of the masticatory muscles and hence 'physiological' in character. It is thought that the physiological and momentary nature of the impulses avoids the stretching and compressing of the periodontal membrane found with the continuous pressure of active appliances. In the functional appliance system the periodontal tissues enjoy periods of rest between impulses and longer rest periods when the activator is out of the mouth, as is usual for a proportion of the 24 hours. The result of this cycle of impulse and resting phase is thought to be a lessening of possible ill effects on the tooth roots and periodontal tissues, tooth movement by activators being characterized by a maintenance of normal periodontal thickness throughout the period of tooth movement (Haupl *et al.*, 1952).

The design and construction of functional appliances

The functional appliance as originally designed was a loose-fitting appliance inserted between the teeth, lying against them at selected points and also making contact with the palate and soft tissues covering the inner side of the mandibular alveolar processes. Through these means functional stimuli were brought to bear on the teeth and through the teeth on the periodontal tissues, alveolar bone and mandibular joint. What is sometimes not quite clear is whether the stimuli applied to the alveolar bone and mandibular joint result from pressures applied to the teeth only or whether it was originally intended to apply stimuli to the alveolar bone through its covering soft tissue also. It is noted by Haupl *et al.* (1952), on the basis of clinical observation, that:

these appliances function even when no longer in contact with the teeth, since the latter had already changed position due to their influence. The results, therefore, were not due to the plate pressing on the teeth.

A fundamental practical and doctrinal consideration concerning the design and use of functional appliances is whether active or pressure elements should or should not be incorporated in the appliances. The principle of functional appliance design and use is that the appliances act through the functional stimuli applied to the teeth, alveolar bone and remoter parts of the dentofacial complex and through the guiding of the teeth during their normal eruption and growth paths. From the doctrinal point of view the addition of active parts to the appliances may be regarded as an illogical complication of the clear fundamental principle of functional stimulation (Watry, 1947). From the purely practical point of view, the addition of active parts to a functional appliance creates technical difficulties in construction and adjustment, and the required looseness of the appliance may lead to imprecision in the application of individual pressures to teeth or may impair the proper functioning of the activator. As, however, teeth may be moved by active pressures, and the vast majority of tooth movements are carried out in this way, if active parts can be incorporated in functional appliances without reducing the efficiency of the appliance as a functional device, there seems to be no real objection to the combination of the two methods of treatment within the same appliance. The true objections to such an amalgamation lie in the possibility that an appliance may be produced that is neither functionally nor actively effective.

The degree to which the scope of a functional appliance may be extended and elaborated by the addition of active parts must lie with the designer and user of the appliance, and when the combination of functional and active pressures in the same appliance becomes too complicated to be efficient, discretion will rule that treatment should be broken down into stages and either active appliances or functional appliances used, depending on the nature of the tooth movements required.

The Andresen appliance

The Andresen appliance or monobloc is probably the most frequently used of the activator group of appliances because of the dramatically successful treatment of Class II division 1 malocclusion that it can effect in some cases. In such cases the true idea of the monobloc as a functional appliance holds good for the reason that the appliance is designed to fit the occlusion only when the mandible and lower dentition are in a forward functional position and the muscular effort used to bring the mandible to its position of centric relation produces the pressures which determine the morphological changes which ensue (*Figure 8.14*).

The use of the monobloc to produce changes in other directions, either a distal shifting of the lower dentition in relation to the upper or changes in lateral direction, is fraught with difficulties which do not arise where the treatment of postnormal occlusion is concerned.

In Class III malocclusion it is not easy to produce such definite functional pressures in the desired directions as it is possible to produce in postnormal occlusion because the mandible cannot be displaced distally in the same way as it can be displaced forwards. The forward position of the mandible used in the functional treatment of postnormal occlusion is a functional position for which there is no equivalent functional distal position in Class III malocclusion.

For the treatment of Class III malocclusion by the Andresen appliance, the best that can be done is to construct an activator which is split horizontally, the two parts being connected by a horizontally-working screw which, when opened, displaces the two portions of the appliance, the lower part distally, the upper mesially by small degrees. When worn as a

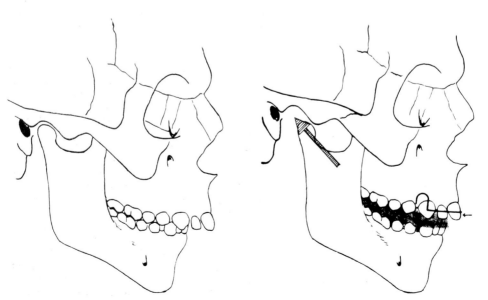

Figure 8.14 The main backward pull of the muscles of mastication is transferred to the teeth individually through the Andresen appliance. The upper teeth are pushed in a distal direction, the lower teeth in a mesial direction

functional appliance, mesial pressure on the upper teeth and distal on the lower can be brought to bear only when the opposing upper and lower dentitions are brought together in a vertical direction by the muscles of mastication and the teeth impinge on the inclined planes in the activator.

The limitations of the activator in the treatment of Class III malocclusion are emphasized by the inclusion in the appliance used in such treatment, by most authorities, of arches or springs intended to bring about proclination of the upper labial segment and retroclination of the teeth in the lower labial segment. Such limited tooth movements in any case often constitute the sole treatment of certain Class III malocclusions, and it may be that these movements could be more effectively carried out by appliances other than the activator equipped with auxiliary bows and springs.

In the treatment of discrepancies in the occlusion in a buccolingual direction, again certain problems are to be found in connection with the use of activator appliances. It is sometimes suggested that different degrees of growth may be brought about in the condyle heads by taking the working bite for an activator with the mandible to one side, so leading to the correction of cross-bite conditions by the wearing of an activator constructed to such a bite. In the treatment of such conditions, however, means are usually shown for producing buccal movement of upper teeth and lingual movement of lower teeth by means of auxiliary attachments on activator appliances.

The success of the Andresen appliance in the treatment of straightforward Class II division 1 malocclusions is a strong recommendation for using the activator only in cases of this kind in the first instance. In restricting the use of the appliance in this way many advantages are to be obtained in that, under favourable circumstances, only one appliance may need to be used, inspections and adjustments may be carried out at relatively infrequent intervals, and at the end of treatment the appliance may simply be discarded or worn once or twice a week for 2–3 months before being discarded. Treatment may be completed within 12 months in favourable cases.

The term 'straightforward Class II division 1 malocclusion' is difficult to define, although what is intended may be comprehensible. The most important considerations are that the dental arches should be well arranged – that is to say, arranged in smooth curves without crowding or impactions in consequence of early loss of deciduous teeth; the upper labial segment may be proclined and spaced, the occlusal relation may be disturbed to the extent of a full unit anteroposteriorly, the overbite may be considerably increased.

Circumstances which indicate doubt as to the advisability of using the Andresen appliance include irregularities of the dental arches following early loss of deciduous teeth or due to disproportion in the size of the teeth and the size of the jaws; breaks in the dental arch following extraction of permanent teeth; open bite due to digit sucking or anomalies of function of the tongue or lips which persist through and after orthodontic treatment; inability of the lips to lie easily in contact when at rest. Such signs suggest difficulties in treatment and are warning signs as to the ultimate stability of the arrangement of the teeth produced in orthodontic treatment by any appliance method. Signs like this indicate that the functional appliance may not be the most suitable apparatus for producing the kinds of tooth rearrangement that are looked for.

It is often advocated that very early treatment of postnormal occlusion using the activator, that is to say, in the deciduous dentition, brings benefits that are not available if treatment is delayed until the permanent dentition is in position. The suggested advantage of beginning treatment very early is that between the time of completion of the deciduous dentition and the accession of the permanent teeth lies a period of active growth and developmental activity in the face, jaws and dentition, and in such conditions the functional type of appliance could be expected to be more effective in directing the development of the occlusion than at a later age. This is theoretically true, and if a number of other important considerations are favourable there is everything to be said for giving the patient the advantages that may come from the utilization of as large a part of the most active growing period of the jaws and dentition as possible. The drawbacks to the very early commencement of orthodontic treatment are that the period of treatment and supervision becomes correspondingly prolonged, with consequent strain on the patient's interest and co-operation; the prolonged wearing of appliances brings its own problems in connection with side-effects arising out of oral hygiene difficulties; the changeover from deciduous to permanent dentition may necessitate a series of new appliances; the occurrence of early loss of deciduous teeth may involve a complicated appliance routine for the patient if space retention and active treatment are continued simultaneously; the later discovery of crowding, when the teeth in the labial segments eventually erupt, may be an unwelcome manifestation, necessitating a revision of the original diagnosis and plan of treatment.

Factors such as these, operating singly or in combination at different times over a prolonged period, can embarrass the course of treatment or nullify the possible benefits of commencing treatment at an early age. There is no clinical control in the individual case to show that early treatment necessarily confers the benefits of a more complete or more stable correction of the occlusal relationship than would be achieved by treatment later on, and it is a known fact that permanent dentitions, complete to the second molar teeth, exhibiting severe degrees of postnormal occlusion, can be quite easily treated by functional appliances to stable, normal occlusal relationship at the age of 11–12 years or older.

The age at which functional treatment of Class II division 1 malocclusion is commenced will be decided in the light of the foregoing considerations.

The construction of the Andresen appliance

The construction of a functional appliance, activator, monobloc or Andresen appliance for the treatment of Class II division 1 malocclusion requires working models and a wax bite. The impressions for the models should be taken in an alginate impression material and the edges of the impressions should extend to the limits of the labial and lingual sulci. It is important to see that the impression extends adequately into the lingual sulcus in the molar region in the lower denture and in the labial sulcus in the upper arch. Impressions that are short in these regions create unnecessary difficulties in the laboratory stages of appliance construction.

As starting points for the making of working bites for the treatment of Class II division 1 malocclusions the following details should be observed:

1. The mandible should be brought forwards until the buccal occlusal relationship is normal anteroposteriorly.

2. The bite should be open to a degree which separates the upper and lower labial segments, making it possible to cover the incisal edges of the lower incisors with the baseplate material of the appliance and leave room for modification of the appliance lingually to the upper incisors.

3. The centre lines should be made to correspond.

The working bite is taken in pink modelling wax, an adequate quantity of which is softened slightly and moulded to a convenient shape which may be varied according to the personal preferences of the operator. A solid transverse block of wax is less likely to become distorted during insertion and removal from the mouth, but may interfere unduly with the patient's tongue and cause difficulty in positioning the mandible. A horseshoe-shaped bite-block is favoured and has the advantage of leaving the lingual area of the mouth free during the taking of the bite, but must be carefully handled during insertion and removal from the mouth as it may easily become warped and hence difficult to place in an accurate position on the working models.

Some of the secrets of taking the working bite include the following points.

Have enough wax in the block and have the main body of wax soft but firm; the surfaces may be flamed just before insertion to ensure a sharp impression of the occlusal surfaces of the teeth. The patient should have something definite to bite on and should not find a completely unresisting mass between the teeth.

The patient should be told what is expected and opening, protrusive, closing and side-to-side movements rehearsed before putting in the bite-block. When actually taking the bite, the patient is told to open, protrude the mandible and close very slowly until told to stop closing, at which point movement should stop with the mandible held quite still. The occlusal relationship can then be checked and any adjustment made by protrusion, retrusion or sideways movement, without opening.

When the occlusal relationship is as required, a very small further closure may be made and the teeth immediately opened. The bite-block should then be removed and chilled in cold water for a minute or so and replaced in the mouth, the patient carefully finding the position of occlusion in the wax. The teeth are then pressed into the wax with gentle firmness and opened. The teeth should come out of the wax with a slight click which indicates that the impression has been confirmed on the fully chilled wax. This second taking of the bite has the advantage of removing any small occlusal obstructions or warps that may have been introduced into the wax when removed from the mouth the first time (*Figures 8.15* and *8.16*).

The working models, which should be at hand, are placed in the working bite and firmly seated. At this stage the correctness and suitability of the bite relationship should be finally checked against the record models and the patient's occlusion. If all is correct, the models should be passed to the laboratory for construction of the appliance (*Figure 8.17*).

As a rule it is not difficult to obtain the working bite for an activator. As the procedure involves a voluntary action on the part of the patient, it is useful to consider patients and their reactions as falling into three categories:

1. The sensible, intelligent patient who understands what is required and can produce the bite relationship that is needed. With such patients the bite may be taken in a moment.

2. The patient who misunderstands what is required but who is over-anxious to help. In such cases much time may be taken up with a large number of incorrect bites and completely spoiled bite-blocks. The more the problem is explained, the more difficult it appears to be to achieve what is required from the patient.

3. The patient who does not understand what is required and who appears unable to carry out any of the movements requested. In such cases it may be possible for the operator to move the mandible into the required position and this may be the best that

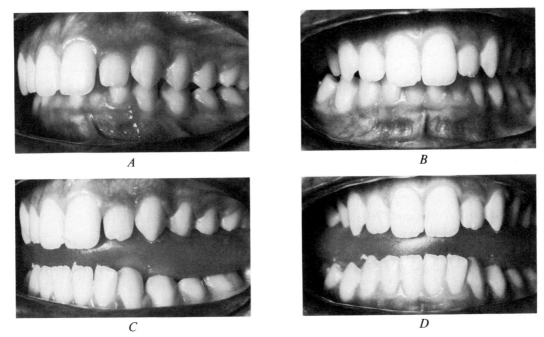

Figure 8.15 *A*, This patient has increased overbite and one unit postnormal occlusion; *B*, the teeth have been opened slightly to show that the centre lines of the upper and lower arches do not correspond; *C*, the bite for an Andresen appliance. The buccal segments are in normal relation anteroposteriorly. The bite has been opened sufficiently to separate the incisors; *D*, the centre lines in the working bite position are made to correspond

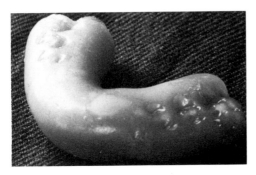

Figure 8.16 The wax bite for constructing the Andresen appliance

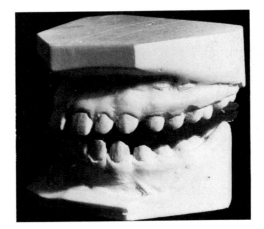

Figure 8.17 Working models placed in wax bite

can be achieved, although with such a low degree of cooperation and understanding on the part of the patient the whole question of treatment with functional appliances in such cases should be carefully considered.

There are very few cases in which serious difficulty arises in taking a bite for the construction of a functional appliance.

Laboratory procedures

An Andresen appliance by tradition is a baseplate which fits both the upper and lower dentitions, with a simple bow which maintains control of the teeth in the upper labial segment.

The Andresen appliance can be constructed by the traditional method using a wax pattern which is flasked and finished in heat-curing acrylic material or the construction can be done using cold-curing acrylic resin.

The traditional method is described here and the cold-curing acrylic method is described in the section dealing with materials used in orthodontics.

Construction of the Andresen appliance using heat-curing acrylic resin takes place in the following stages – articulating the models; construction of the labial bow; waxing the baseplates; inserting the labial bow; joining the baseplates together; flasking, packing and finishing.

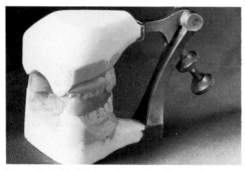

Figure 8.18 Models have been placed on a plane-line articulator. The blades of the articulator are parallel

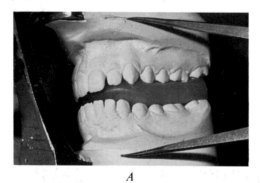

A

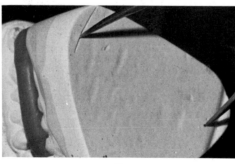

C

Articulating the models

The easiest way of articulating the models is to use a standard, plane-line articulator and fix the casts with the incisor teeth facing towards the hinge of the articulator. The lingual aspect of the models faces outwards and this greatly facilitates the waxing up of the baseplate (*Figure 8.18*). It is important to have the bases cut down enough to permit the insertion of the models, with the intervening working bite, between the blades or forks of the articulator when they are parallel. It is then possible to withdraw the casts from the articulator without separating them from the working bite or from the waxed-up appliance when this later stage is finished. The possibility of removing the models from the articulator in this way avoids damage to the plaster teeth which might occur if the articulated models are simply opened from the wax bite or from the waxed-up appliance. If the models are taken off the articulator together they may be separated from the wax bite by slight warming, if necessary, and the waxed appliance may be gently eased off prior to flasking and finishing the appliance.

When the models are fixed on the articulator the setting screw is locked, and as a further precaution the vertical dimension is measured and registered on the bottom of the lower model before the models are disturbed from their positions in the wax bite (*Figure 8.19*).

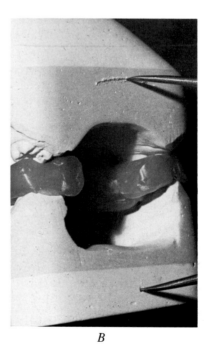

B

Figure 8.19 The height of the bite is measured; *A*, anteriorly, *B*, posteriorly; *C*, the measurement is recorded on the base of the models

Construction of the labial bow

The models are removed from the articulator and freed from the wax bite and from any particles of wax that may be adhering to them.

A plain labial bow is then constructed for the upper model extending distally to the centres of the labial surfaces of the canine teeth and with a U-loop at either side. The ends of the bow pass between the canine and first premolar teeth into the palate. The bow should be made of a robust gauge of hard stainless steel wire of about 0.9 mm thickness. If a more resilient bow is required, a thickness of 0.8 mm may be used, in which case it is advisable to reinforce the wire at the point where it enters the baseplate by sliding on a short length of annealed stainless steel tube of the correct internal diameter (*Figure 8.20*). The thinner wire will be required if pressure is to be exerted on the upper incisor teeth by compressing the U-loops, as bows of the kind described are always relatively stiff and it is difficult to obtain sensitive control of the amount of pressure exerted by bows made of rather thick wires. The labial bow as described is used to cause the teeth in the labial segment to follow the movement of the teeth in the buccal segments as changes in the occlusal relation take place. The bow may also be activated a little to produce a lingual inclination of the teeth in the labial segment.

When bringing the ends of the labial bow through into the palate of the upper model, it is important to keep the wire clear of the teeth and to make the tags pass equidistantly between the upper and lower rows of teeth. Sometimes the tags are brought through to the palate in contact with the embrasure between the upper canine and first premolar teeth. In consequence, when the appliance is later trimmed with a steel bur there is danger of damaging the wire as it lies near the surface of the baseplate material. If the wire is passed midway between the upper and lower teeth it is deep within the baseplate material

in this situation and the risk is less of cutting as far down as the wire when trimming the appliance.

The final anchorage of the ends of the labial bow in the baseplate can be quite simple, and if the tips of the ends are turned down against the palate this will ensure that the tag is held securely in the baseplate material.

Waxing the baseplates

This should be done in the following stages:

1. Wax up the upper and lower baseplates.
2. Insert the labial bow in the upper baseplate.
3. Join the baseplates together with the models on the articulator.
4. Smooth off the waxing of the complete appliance.

When the time comes to transform the wax prototype of the appliance into acrylic material this may be done in one of two ways. Either the wax may be sealed to the working casts on which it was constructed and models and wax embedded in the flask for completion of the packing and polymerizing procedures; or the wax image of the appliance may be removed from the plaster casts on which it was constructed and embedded in the flask by itself and subsequently converted into an acrylic reproduction.

The second procedure is the simpler and more satisfactory, but it is essential that the wax pattern of the appliance should reproduce accurately the fitting surfaces of the teeth and gingival margins of the casts on which it was constructed, and care must be taken to ensure that the wax pattern is not allowed to warp.

In waxing-up the upper and lower baseplates, therefore, it is essential to see that the wax is soft enough to take a good impression of the embrasures between the lingual aspects of the teeth.

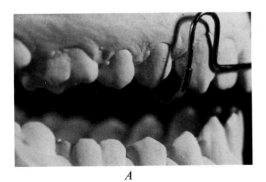
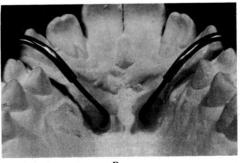

| A | B |

Figure 8.20 *A*, The labial bow of 0.8 mm wire is reinforced with stainless steel tubing where it will enter the baseplate. Note that the tag of the bow runs well clear of the upper canine and premolar teeth; *B*, the tags of the labial bow are turned down at right angles to the palate. This simple attachment is perfectly satisfactory

The recommended procedure is to wet the dental casts in fairly warm water, but not to soak the plaster so long that free water remains lying on the surface when the models are left for a few moments in the air. The wetting and slight warming of the casts have two objects. First, wax will not stick to the damp surface and secondly, the slightly warm plaster will not chill the soft wax and prevent it from spreading into the gingival crevices.

To adapt the wax to the tooth surfaces and the adjoining gingiva it is better to apply the wax as a roll about 1 cm in diameter with a well-softened outer layer.

This roll is curved to fit the dental arch lingually, lying just below the gum margin (*Figure 8.21*). The soft surface is then pressed out against the teeth and into the embrasures between them and on to their occlusal surfaces (*Figure 8.22*). It is necessary to work quickly when doing this initial adaptation of the wax. Care must be taken in the incisor region not to break off any of the teeth. If the wax is soft, light but sufficient pressure employed, and as a precaution, the incisor teeth supported on the labial side with a curved forefinger, there will be no danger of breaking the teeth.

In the lower model the softened wax should be taken up to and over the incisal edges of the front teeth in a thin layer. It is important to avoid putting a thick layer of hard wax over the lower incisors at this stage, as when the baseplates are subsequently pressed into contact a spot of excessive pressure may occur over the lower incisors, leading to fracture of the plaster teeth (*Figure 8.23*).

When the wax has been adapted to the teeth and gum margins the remainder of the roll should be used for the construction of the baseplate areas of the upper and lower parts of the appliance. In the upper arch the wax may be stretched down into the palate and the segments from either side joined in the midline with a hot wax knife. It is important to avoid pulling the wax away from the teeth. If there is sufficient wax in the roll this method has the advantage that the upper part of the appliance is made in one piece of wax. If there is surplus wax, the palate area should be scraped down to a suitable and uniform thickness and smoothed with the flame. If necessary, wax can be added to complete the construction of the palate.

An alternative method for the completion of the construction of the upper baseplate is as follows. When the wax has been well adapted to the teeth it may be scraped down from the lingual aspect until only what is essential to fit the teeth and gum margin is left, after which a palate may be added as a single layer of softened wax. With this method it may be difficult to avoid leaving a noticeable line of junction between the two wax applications when the appliance is seen from the palatal aspect, and in scraping down the first application of wax great care

must be exercised to avoid going too far and taking a cut off an underlying tooth.

In the lower arch the wax roll is usually sufficient to complete the construction of the baseplate; the wax is simply pressed down into the lingual sulcus and trimmed to shape.

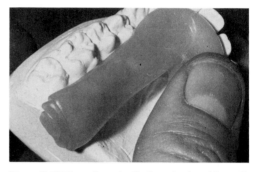

Figure 8.21 The softened roll of wax is placed lingually and just below the level of the occlusal surfaces of the teeth

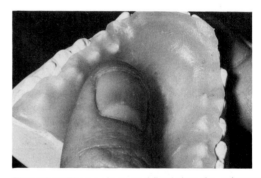

Figure 8.22 The wax is pressed firmly into the embrasures between the teeth and spread down into the palate

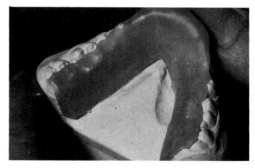

Figure 8.23 The lower baseplate waxed up from a roll of softened wax. Note that the incisal edges of the front teeth are capped with a thin layer of wax

Inserting the labial bow

The simplest method for placing the labial bow in the upper baseplate is to soften the appropriate area of the baseplate with a hot knife sufficiently to tack in the bow in its required position. The softened wax is cooled with an air stream and the bow fastened with pink wax flowed around the tags. The method of heating the tags of the bow and melting them into the baseplate is clumsy and liable to be inaccurate as it is difficult to heat the tags to the right temperature for long enough to give time to place the wire precisely. If the wire is not hot enough it will not melt the wax. If it is too hot an excessive amount of wax is melted and runs away, after which there is a delay while the wax cools enough to hold the wire; meanwhile, the bow must be held in place with great accuracy. The fact that the recommended fitting of the tags requires that they do not lie against the plaster, but only touch at their bent-down ends, means that the bow can usually be held in position by the turned down tips for positioning purposes, after which the bow is properly secured with wax flowed around the tags, fastening them to the surface of the baseplate (*Figure 8.24*).

Joining the baseplates together

The models are replaced on the articulator and the articulator closed. At this stage it is important to examine the occluding surfaces of the two plates to make quite sure that they do not actually touch, but that there is at least 1 mm clearance between the wax overlying the occlusal and incisal surfaces of the teeth. The reason for this clearance is that when softened wax is put between the models and the baseplates pressed together, there is a risk that if the baseplates touch at any point, excessive pressure at this spot may damage the underlying plaster, particularly in the incisor area.

The sealing together of the baseplates is done with a roll of very well-softened wax, the occlusal surfaces of the baseplates being flamed just before inserting the roll and closing the articulator.

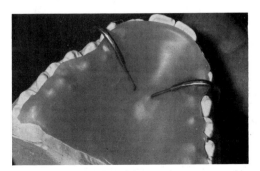

Figure 8.24 The labial bow is waxed in position

When the articulator is being closed a check should be made on the vertical dimension between the upper and lower models, using the registration marks and recorded dimension originally provided. Care should be taken to see that the articulator is closed as far as, but not beyond, the original registration.

The waxing-up of the appliance is completed by smoothing off the joint between the upper and lower parts, attending to the fit and neatness of the waxing around the incisor segments, and smoothing the lingual surface of the appliance with a small fine flame of the blowlamp. The wax is then thoroughly chilled in cold water or left in a cold atmosphere until cold right through. The models are removed together from the articulator and then each model is very carefully taken off the wax appliance. Final trimming of the appliance may then be carried out; the lateral flanges may be reduced to half the width of the teeth in the buccal segments as this will save considerable time and labour in cutting the finished appliance; the lingual flange of the lower part of the appliance can be trimmed to the correct depth and smoothed and rounded. No other trimming of the appliance should be done at this stage. The models should then be finally seated in the appliance to ensure that no occlusal interferences have been introduced through the trimming of the buccal flanges, and the wax appliance is ready for flasking and finishing (*Figure 8.25*).

Flasking, packing and finishing

The wax pattern of the appliance is flasked upside down in the deep part of the flask with the plaster brought to the posterior edge of the palate and the lower edge of the lingual flange of the lower baseplate (*Figure 8.26*).

During the flasking process a thin mix of the plaster should be brushed into the impression of the various tooth surfaces in the wax to ensure that air bubbles are not trapped. A wetting agent should also be used.

This method of investment ensures that the fitting surface of the appliance is in one half of the flask so that distorting the appliance during packing and pressing the flask is avoided. The second half of the flask is poured after applying separating medium to the lower half. When the plaster is set the flask is heated and the halves separated, the wax washed out, the flask packed and the baseplate material processed in the normal way. The acrylic materials in the pink colour are perfectly satisfactory.

After processing and cooling, the appliance is deflasked, cleaned and dried. Excess acrylic material, present as 'flash' around the lower and posterior edges, is removed and the appliance smoothed and polished. At this stage the acrylic appliance is placed on the models which are

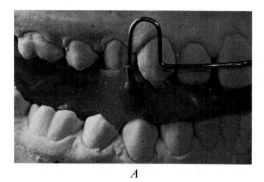
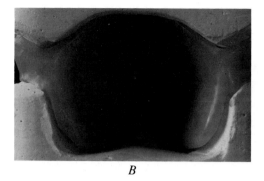

A   *B*

Figure 8.25 *A*, The completed waxed-up Andresen appliance; *B*, the lingual view of the appliance. Note that the lingual undercuts in the molar region of the lower model have been plastered out and that in this area the appliance is constructed with well-rounded flanges against which the tongue lies comfortably

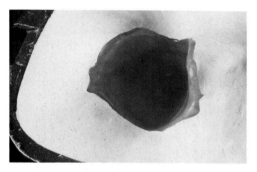

Figure 8.26 The Andresen appliance embedded in the deep half of the flask. The appliance is packed from the lingual side

baseplate material should be removed lingually to the upper incisors, distally to the teeth in the upper buccal segments, and mesially to the teeth in the lower buccal segments. The capping over the lower incisors should be left in position (*Figure 8.27*). Trimming is best done with a steel bone bur in the straight handpiece, and if the facets which must be left in the buccal segments are marked with a soft

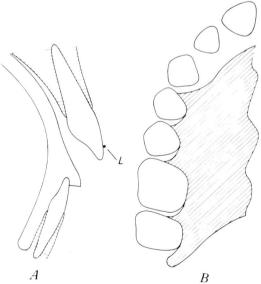

A   *B*

Figure 8.27 *A*, The trimming of the Andresen appliance in the incisor region. Baseplate material is removed behind the upper incisors well up to the apical region. The lower incisors remain capped in the baseplate; *L* is the labial bow; *B*, the trimming of the Andresen appliance in the upper buccal segments. Note that the appliance impinges on the mesial aspects of the premolar and molar teeth and is cut away behind the labial segment. In the lower arch the facets are made to touch the teeth in the buccal segments distally

returned to the articulator and registration of the vertical dimension checked. The appliance should fit the occlusion of the patient exactly with the mandible forwards in the working bite position.

Fitting and adjusting of the activator

The activator is placed in the mouth exactly as it is received from the laboratory. If the teeth do not meet evenly and exactly in their impressions in the appliance, anteriorly and posteriorly, and there is any sign that the bite has been 'raised' or otherwise disturbed during the construction of the appliance, the appliance should be reconstructed as it never is possible to make an ill-fitting appliance fit satisfactorily by cutting or otherwise adjusting it.

Cutting the activator

If the appliance fits correctly it should then be cut to facilitate the tooth movements that are intended. The cutting of an Andresen appliance means that

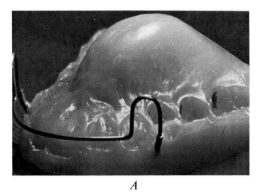
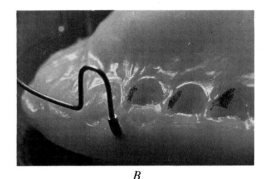

A *B*

Figure 8.28 *A*, The completed Andresen appliance; *B*, the areas intended as facets to impinge on the teeth in the buccal segments have been marked with lead pencil

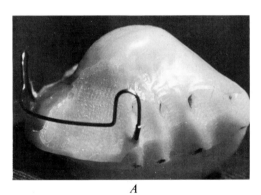
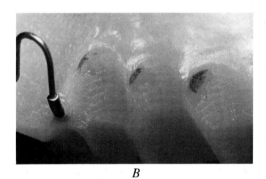

A *B*

Figure 8.29 *A*, The Andresen appliance after the left side has been trimmed in the incisor region and in the buccal segments; *B*, the pencil markings on the facets are still to be seen. Note the channels along which eruption of the teeth can take place

lead pencil before cutting is started, the trimming may be done with great precision (*Figure 8.28*). The channels which run between the upper and lower teeth in the buccal segments should run downwards and backwards (*Figure 8.29*). If it is intended that there should be expansion of the buccal segments, the channels in the appliance may be constructed to guide the premolar and molar teeth buccally (*Figure 8.30*). In these circumstances the buccal movement of the teeth can only take place if the teeth erupt farther.

Any sharp edges left by the cutting of the appliance are smoothed off and all is ready for final trial of the appliance in the mouth.

Case reports

A.C., aged 12 years (*Figure 8.31*).

Diagnosis

Dental base relation a little postnormal. Upper lip a little short, lower lip postures lingually to the upper incisors. The dental arches were complete with the permanent teeth to the first permanent molars, the upper incisors were proclined and spaced, the lower incisors were well aligned. The lower buccal segments were one unit postnormal to the upper, the overbite was increased and complete. The right upper first molar occluded lingually to the lower first molar (*Figure 8.31A*).

Treatment

A Sved plate was worn for 3 months as an experiment in patient cooperation. The overbite was reduced and there was a slight improvement in the occlusal relation. An Andresen appliance was then

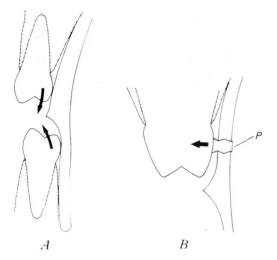

A   *B*

Figure 8.30 *A*, If required, the channels in which the buccal teeth lie are curved outwards, so guiding the eruption of these teeth and creating expansion of the arches; *B*, buccal movement of a molar tooth by means of a pad of rubber (*P*) pulled into an undercut hole in the baseplate. The plug should project about 1–2 mm against the tooth and should be cut off flush on the lingual side. The rubber used is separating rubber which is in strips about 3 mm square in section

fitted. Cephalometric X-rays and record models were made. Eighteen months later the occlusal relation was correct anteroposteriorly. The incisor relation had improved very greatly. The relationship of right upper first molar to the lower was corrected by means of a rubber plug pulled into the appliance lingually to the upper molar (Hopkin, 1958) (*Figure 8.30B*). A Hawley retainer with inclined plane was fitted and worn for 6 months. Final records were taken 1 year after completion of the treatment with the Andresen appliance.

Table 8.1 details the cephalometric measurements before and after treatment. From this it can be seen that SNA–SNB difference had hardly changed. The upper incisors were retroclined by 22°, the lower incisors proclined 6°. Both upper and lower prognathism was slightly less after than before treatment.

Figure 8.32A and *B* shows casts before and after treatment of a classic Class II division 1 malocclusion with regular dental arches and proclination and spacing of the upper anterior teeth. The third molars were absent, the lips were potentially competent. Dental base relationship was slightly postnormal. The patient was treated over a period of 18 months and normal occlusion was produced with retroclination of the upper incisors and lip seal at rest. The new occlusal relationship has remained stable (*Figure 8.32C* and *D*).

Table 8.1 Cephalometric analysis

	Before	*After*	*Difference*
SNA	78.0°	76.0°	−2.0°
SNB	74.5°	73.0°	−1.5°
SNA–SNB difference	3.5°	3.0°	−0.5°
Upper central incisors to SN	122°	100°	−22°
Lower central incisors to mandibular plane	89°	95°	+6°

Figure 8.33 shows a patient aged 13 years with classic Class II division 1 malocclusion with a full dentition up to the second permanent molars present and with considerable spacing and scissors bite on the first premolars. Dental base relationship was postnormal and the lips potentially competent (*Figure 8.33A–C*).

The patient was treated with an Andresen appliance and the condition responded rapidly and favourably, the occlusal and incisor relationships became corrected and lip posture became normal. There was some spacing between the labial and the buccal segments in the upper arch which it was hoped to use to improve the incisor relationship further, but the patient was so gratified with the improvement to date that she ceased attending for supervision and appeals to keep any further appointments fell on deaf ears (*Figure 8.33D–F*).

Figure 8.34 shows the records of a patient aged 12 years having individually excellent dental arches but with one unit postnormal occlusion, postnormal dental base relationship, low Frankfort/mandibular angle and competent lip posture. Both the upper and the lower incisors were proclined and there was a considerable degree of spacing. There was also scissors bite on all the premolars (*Figure 8.34A–D*).

The malocclusion was treated with expansion of the lower arch, extra-oral traction to the upper arch with extraction of the second molars and a final period of treatment with an Andresen appliance (*Figure 8.34E–H*).

The Bionator

The Bionator appliance described by Balters (1952, 1965) has recently enjoyed a resurgence of interest and is currently gaining in popularity over the Andresen appliance in the treatment of Class II division 1 malocclusion. The principles which the Bionator embraces are fundamentally the same as those of the Andresen appliance. To some extent, however, it occupies a position between the Activator and Function Regulator in that Balters emphasizes the role of the orofacial muscles, in particular the tongue and buccinator muscles, in the

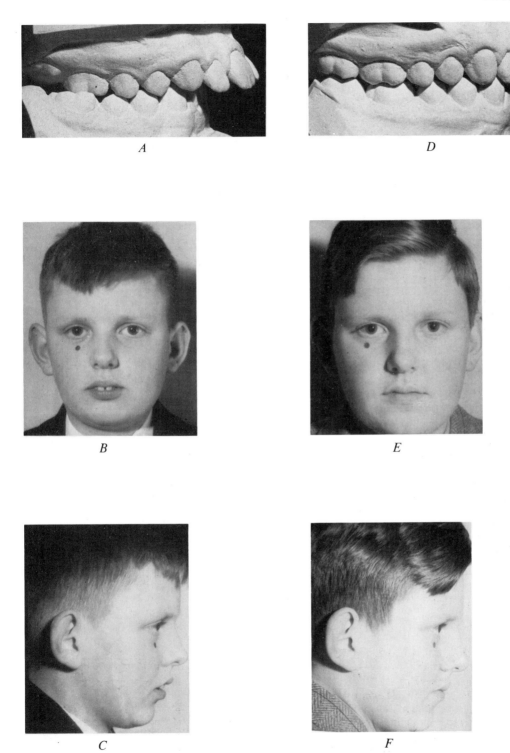

A

D

B

E

C

F

Figure 8.31 Postnormal occlusion with lingual occlusion of the right upper first molar. The condition was treated with an Andresen appliance and the upper molar was moved buccally by means of a rubber plug pulled into a hole drilled in the Andresen appliance; *A–C*, before treatment; *D–F*, after treatment

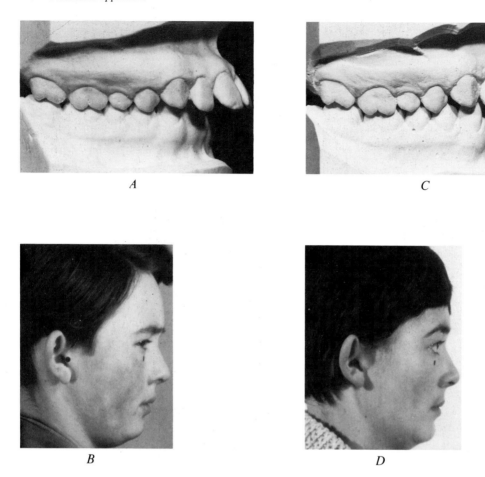

A

C

B

D

Figure 8.32 The classical Class II division 1 malocclusion treated with an Andresen appliance over a period of 18 months; *A* and *B*, before treatment; *C* and *D*, after treatment. The final record was taken when the patient was 18 years of age

aetiology of malocclusion. Consequently, alteration of tongue posture and screening of the buccal segments from the influence of the buccinator are seen as important components of treatment with this appliance (*Figure 8.35*).

From the practical point of view, the great advantage of the Bionator over the Andresen is that the Bionator is 'open', i.e. much of the acrylic resin which characterizes the Andresen has been eliminated or replaced by wire, giving the Bionator a more skeletal appearance. The acrylic elements applied to the lower incisor and buccal teeth have been retained and the two halves are connected palatally by a modified Coffin spring constructed from 1.25 mm wire. The 0.9 mm labial bow is recurved in the buccal segments to prevent the cheeks from interposing between the upper and lower buccal teeth, thus impeding their eruption. The clinical

benefits of these modifications are that the appliance is considerably less bulky than the Andresen which permits it to be worn up to 24 hours per day, being removed only for meals and cleaning and enabling wear to continue even when mouth breathing is enforced by temporary nasal obstruction.

The working bite is taken in a similar manner to that for the Andresen appliance, except that in an anteroposterior direction, an edge-to-edge relationship is aimed at. In cases with excessively large overjets this may need to be achieved in two stages. As with the Andresen, the bite should be sufficiently open to allow the lower incisors to be capped with acrylic resin.

The stages in construction of the Bionator are shown in *Figure 8.36*.

Clinical experience with the appliance has shown

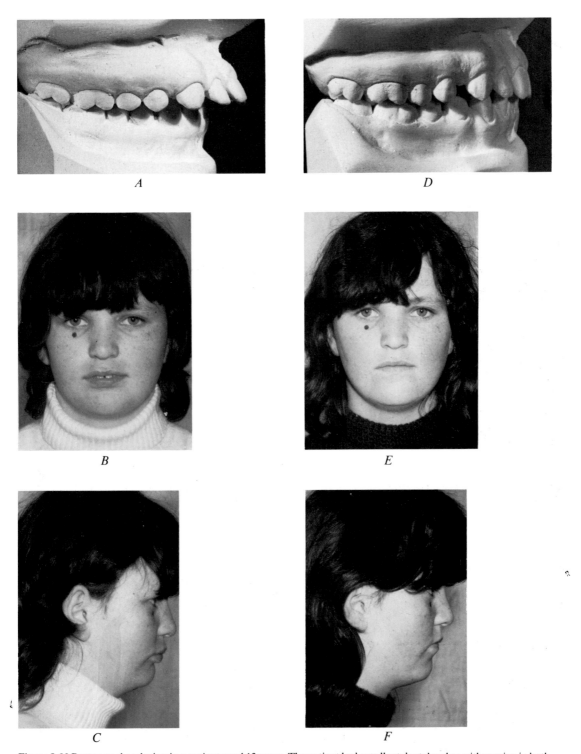

Figure 8.33 Postnormal occlusion in a patient aged 13 years. The patient had excellent dental arches with spacing in both upper and lower labial segments. Treatment was started with an Andresen appliance and the condition rapidly improved. The patient was so pleased that she discontinued treatment before it was fully complete; *A–C*, before treatment; *D–F*, after treatment

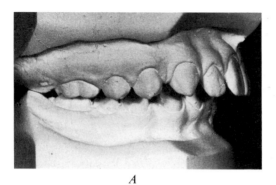

A

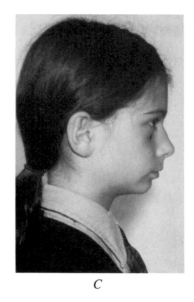

C

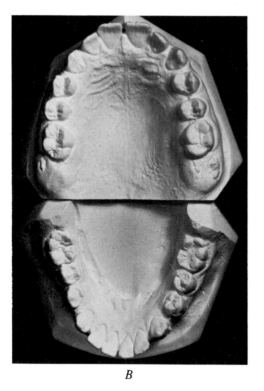

B

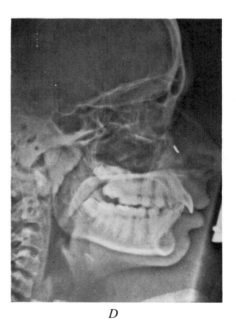

D

Figure 8.34 A patient aged 12 years with postnormal occlusion, low Frankfort/mandibular and maxillo/mandibular angles, proclined lower incisors and scissors bite of the premolars. Tongue and lip posture and function were normal. Treatment was by expanding the lower arch, extraction of the upper second molars and using extra-oral traction to the upper arch with a removable traction appliance. Treatment was completed with an Andresen appliance; *A–D*, before treatment; *E–H*, after treatment

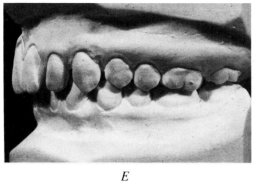

E

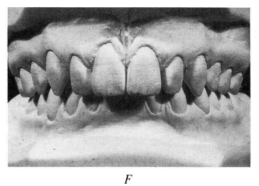

F

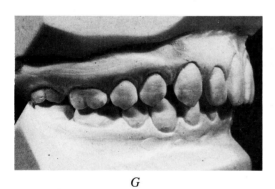

G

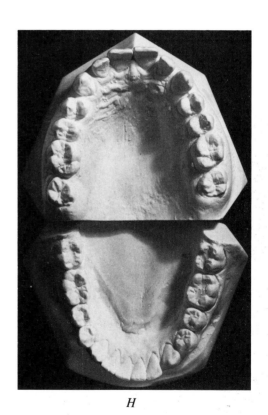

H

Figure 8.34 continued

that the lower lingual acrylic section is prone to breakage and this may be avoided by splitting the appliance in the midline and joining the two halves with 0.7 mm stress-breaking wire.

The buccal acrylic facets are trimmed in a manner similar to that described for the Andresen appliance. This permits the premolars and molars to be

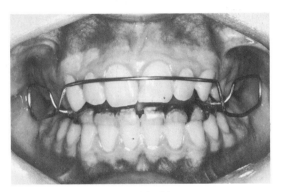

Figure 8.35 Intra-oral view of the Bionator

guided into their optimum positions. Where deciduous teeth are present, the lingual halves of their crowns should remain covered with acrylic resin to improve the stability of the appliance. When the deciduous molars are shed, the acrylic is removed to facilitate eruption of the premolars.

Balters has also described two further variants of the appliance which may be used in the treatment of open bite and Class III malocclusion.

Case reports

Figure 8.37 illustrates the treatment of a severe Class II division 1 malocclusion.

Diagnosis

The patient, a girl aged 10 years 1 month presented with a discrepancy in ANB of 10° and overjet of 12 mm. Early loss of deciduous teeth masked the fact that the lower arch was basically slightly crowded and there was slight crowding of the upper incisors. The lips were incompetent, the lower lip resting against the incisal edge of the upper incisor.

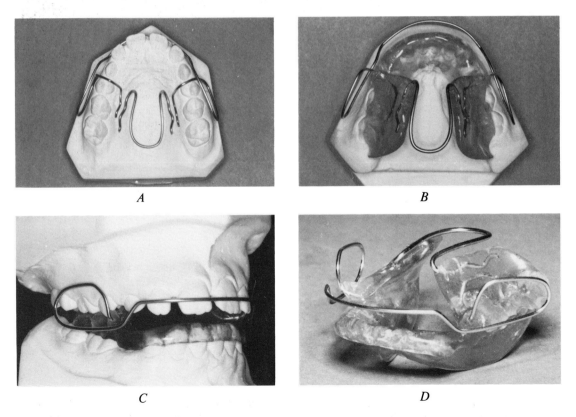

A

B

C

D

Figure 8.36 *A*, Occlusal view of maxillary wire elements; *B*, occlusal view of the completed appliance on the mandibular cast; *C* and *D*, the finished appliance on and off the articulator

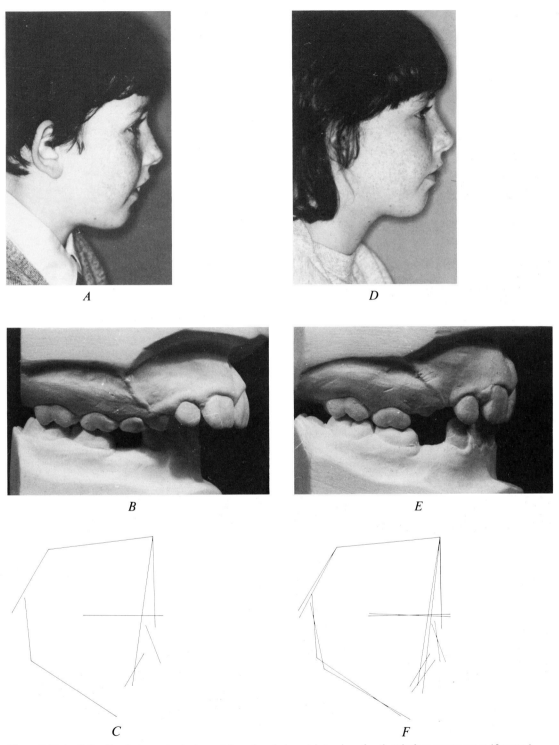

A

D

B

E

C

F

Figure 8.37 *A–C*, Profile photograph, study models and cephalometric tracing of patient before treatment at 10 years 1 month; *D* and *E*, profile photographs and study models at 11 years 7 months pending the eruption of successional teeth and completion of treatment; *F*, cephalometric tracings before and after Bionator treatment superimposed on S–N, registered at S (10 years 1 month/11 years 7 months)

Treatment

The presence of crowding meant that functional therapy could only be considered as the first phase of treatment but this was deemed necessary because of the risk of trauma to the upper incisors if left untreated at this stage. Early interception of the malocclusion might also ameliorate the unfavourable soft-tissue posture and skeletal relationship and aesthetic improvement at this stage could but encourage the patient.

As the inclination of the lower incisors was normal, a Bionator appliance was chosen in preference to a Fränkel I appliance which tends to produce some proclination of the lower incisors.

Good cooperation in wearing the appliance was obtained, the buccal segment relationship being corrected to normal and the overjet to 3 mm in 7 months. Maximal wear was continued for a further 3 months and subsequently reduced to night only pending the eruption and extraction of the first premolars and completion of treatment with fixed appliances.

A second cephalogram taken 18 months later at 11 years 7 months showed a reduction of ANB of 3° brought about largely by an increase in SNB in conjunction with no change in SNA. The lower incisor inclination was virtually unchanged while the upper incisors had tipped lingually by 16°. The upper incisors were now within control of the lower lip although the lips remained incompetent.

The function corrector

This appliance was originally referred to as the 'Function Corrector' by its originator and is also known as the 'Function Regulator', but the term most widely used now is 'The Fränkel Appliance' or, more briefly, the F.R. 1, 2 or 3. The appliance was originated by Dr Rolf Fränkel of Zwickau, East Germany, about the middle of the present century.

The basic theoretical principle underlying the mode of action of this appliance is the idea that within the jaws and dentoalveolar processes there is, at practically every site, the possibility of bone deposition and resorption, especially during the growing period. It is further held that the amounts and directions of bone deposition are influenced by variations in the pressure environment of the jaws and alveolar processes brought about by the posture and activity of the tongue, lips and cheeks. The function corrector, therefore, seeks to modify the soft-tissue positions and activities and thereby to influence the amounts and directions of bone deposition that are taking place within the dento-alveolar complex.

Function correctors are shields which lie in the vestibule of the mouth and stand clear of all portions of the dentoalveolar system which are under-developed. The wire elements unite the lateral shields with the lip pads and serve also as guiding, stabilizing and reflex-inducing factors.

It is from the physical nature of the appliance and its theoretical mode of action that the appliance derives its name, 'The Vestibular Appliance or Function Corrector'.

The following extract from the writings of Dr Fränkel embodies what appear to be the main theoretical principles which underlie the mode of action of the appliance and determine its application to the treatment of various kinds of irregularities and malocclusions.

Configuration and structure of the tooth-bearing gnathic skeleton are subject to mechanical influences of the environment which have the effect of modifying the growth sites and leading to the formation of a supporting structure. Such mechanical modification and activation of the growth sites may be due to the following four types of factors:

1. Mechanical factors which are associated with the development, i.e. the influence of growth-linked changes in the size and shape of skeletal and environmental soft tissues.
2. Mechanical factors of a functional nature, i.e. the influence of physical functions such as oral seal, mastication, deglutition, play of features, respiration and so on.
3. The mechanical potential of the atmospheric pressure which by acting on the soft tissue mass is responsible, to a considerable extent, for the mechanical situation in the gnathic region.
4. The potential of the force of gravity, which exerts its influence especially on the tongue and the mandible.

It should therefore be the chief aim of orthodontic therapy to trace and eliminate any abnormal mechanical potentials in the environmental soft tissues. Mechanical factors of a functional nature are the most serious of those mentioned above, and any dysfunction or complete absence of oral seal deserves our closest attention.

In dealing with this we should bear in mind the fact that a physiologically normal oral seal is only ensured if three requirements are fulfilled:

1. Anterior oral seal, brought about by lip seal with normal tension.
2. Posterior oral seal, brought about by the contact between soft palate and root of the tongue.
3. Median oral seal, brought about by the contact between dorsum of the tongue and hard palate.

In this connection I would refer to the investigations made by Donders (quoted by Eckert-Möbius, 1953), Körbitz (1914), Noltemeier (1949), Eckert-Möbius (1962) and Fränkel (1964). According to these authors, the natural rest position of the tongue against the roof of the palate is not due to muscular action but is maintained solely by the action of the atmospheric pressure. Their investigations revealed that the deglutition reflex, which is accompanied by lip seal, results in the air being 'pumped out' of the cavum proprium by the tongue's peristalsis, thus creating a partial vacuum which is completely filled by the soft tissue of the tongue, under the action of the atmospheric pressure. In this way we get a completely enclosed space between tongue on the one hand and lips and cheeks on the other hand.

This space must be regarded as the most appropriate site for directing the morphogenesis of the tooth-bearing alveolar process.

But the above-mentioned environmental mechanical factors and their importance for the morphogenesis and configuration of the gnathic skeleton should not be interpreted in terms of functional influences alone. The neuromotor functions of respiration, food intake and digestion are not acquired, like motor functions, but are congenital, that is to say, they are perfect from birth owing to the unconditioned reflex control mechanism. This functional mechanism therefore is a hereditary feature. Moreover, the individual and hereditary characteristics become clearly evident in the play of the features and in this respect one may say that, given a normal environment, its mechanical influences assume the quality of genetic information. Thus the genotypical arrangement of the soft tissue and its neuromotor functions affords an excellent explanation for all cases of striking family likeness. But as the phenotype invariably constitutes a combination of hereditary and environmental factors the appearance of orofacial soft tissue and especially the play of the features should not be taken merely as the result of a hereditary disposition.

They should also be regarded as the reflection of the individual's psychic development, which results from his confrontation with the environment. This is the background which gave rise to our optimistic view that any soft-tissue atypia will be amenable to functional treatment.

If we subscribe to the principle of a 'proper education of the jaw', an analysis of the above will show that the first and foremost object of orthodontics should be a normalization of the environment of the growing jaw. Our therapeutic measures should chiefly be directed at eliminating any atypical features in the threefold oral seal and acquired habits, especially any abnormal functioning of the perioral muscles during deglutition. Normalization of the oral seal also creates the main prerequisites for a normalization of respiration.

Teleradiographic examinations showed that this kind of treatment resulted frequently in a significant dilatation of the epipharynx and recession of the swelling of the nasopharyngeal tonsil.

The function corrector has been shown to be an effective appliance for the treatment of malocclusions of certain kinds and where such malocclusions are encountered the use of the function corrector should be considered.

Malocclusions of the Class II division 1 and Class III type and anterior open bite have reacted favourably to treatment in the authors' experience.

Design of the function corrector

There are three types of function corrector.

Type I function corrector or F.R.1

This type is used in the treatment of Angle Class I and Class II division 1 malocclusions.

The lower lip shields are supports for the lower lip and prevent the action of the mentalis muscle in producing pressure on the lower incisors. The function of the lower lip shields is valuable in situations where there is retroclination or crowding of the lower incisors whether the occlusion as a whole is normal or postnormal.

The buccal shields relieve pressure on the lateral aspects of the dental arches which leads to expansion, especially in the upper arch.

In Class II division 1 cases the lower lip shield encourages a forward position of the lower lip which embraces the shield on closing the lips.

The action of the U-loops in the lingual bow is important in the reduction of distocclusion. If the lower jaw slips back from the protruded position in which the regulator is made, the U-loops on the lingual bow make contact with the mucous membrane on the lingual surface on the lower anterior alveolar tissues, thereby initiating a reflex which encourages the lower jaw to adopt the forward position.

In the treatment of postnormal occlusion, whether division 1 or 2, a forward positioning of the lower jaw in taking the functional bite is necessary.

The F.R.1 appliance is also used in the treatment of open bite. When used for this purpose, Fränkel advises that lip pads should be placed below both the upper and the lower lips and states that it is not necessary to place any screen or wire to limit the projection of the tongue between the incisor teeth.

Type II function corrector or F.R.2

This is used for treatment of Class II division 2 malocclusion, and retroclination of the upper incisors is dealt with by a lingual arch in the upper part of the appliance behind the upper incisors. Activation of this arch will produce proclination of these teeth. Otherwise, the action of the corrector is the same as in Class II division 1 types of cases in that the labial pads at the lower incisors relieve pressure of the lower lip on the lower incisors, and the correct occlusal relation is established by the bite with which the appliance is made.

Type III function corrector or F.R.3

In this type the pressure of the upper lip on the upper incisors is relieved by pads which are placed over the upper alveolar process, and the action of the labial bow on the lower part of the appliance has the effect of correcting the incisor relationship, if necessary, by the retroclination of the lower incisors.

Construction of the function corrector

Clinical procedures

Impressions are taken in alginate material of the upper and lower dental arches and adjacent tissues. The impressions must extend to the full depth of the buccal and lingual sulci and cover the palate to the posterior limit of the hard palate. The impressions are poured in a hard or stone plaster and the working casts should be at hand when the bite is being taken.

An adequate roll of softened pink wax is used and the nature of the bite registration will vary with the type of malocclusion being treated. The molar part of the bite must be adequately registered (*Figure 8.38*).

In Class I malocclusion, the bite is taken with the incisors edge-to-edge and in contact.

In Class II malocclusion (divisions 1 and 2), when taking the bite, the mandible is moved forwards to bring the buccal segments into a normal antero-posterior relationship and the teeth are closed together into contact. The amount by which the mandible is moved forwards is influenced also to some extent by the overjet and overbite and inclination of the incisor segments. The comfort of the patient when wearing the appliance must be considered and to bring the mandible too far forwards will mean that the appliance may not be worn.

In Class III malocclusion, the bite is taken as nearly as possible with the incisors edge-to-edge, no protrusion of the mandible being allowed. It is sometimes advisable not to close the teeth fully together into contact if the lower incisors overlap the upper to any marked degree and, when constructing the appliance, to place bite-blocks between the upper and lower buccal segments attached to the buccal screens. Such bite-planes or blocks prop the bite open sufficiently to allow the upper incisors to procline without the obstruction of the lower incisor teeth. If the lower incisor teeth do not overlap the uppers it is not usually necessary to put bite-propping planes in the buccal segments.

Laboratory procedures

The following notes apply to the construction of an F.R.1 appliance.

1. The working casts are mounted on a plain articulator using the working wax bite. The lower labial sulcus on the working model is trimmed with a round vulcanite cutter to ensure that the sulcus is sufficiently deep. If the impression does not record the full depth of the labial sulcus in the lower incisor region the labial pads when constructed will not hold the lower lip away from the lower incisor teeth. Even if the sulcus is deepened too much the labial pads which result can be trimmed to prevent irritation of the labial sulcus, but pads which are too shallow cannot easily be added to at a later stage.

2. In the buccal segments wax of the thickness of 1.5 mm is placed over the buccal segments of the teeth and the adjacent mucosal covering of the alveolar process. When the buccal screens are subsequently constructed they will then be clear of the teeth and soft tissues.

3. The wire work, consisting of the following parts, is constructed in 0.9 mm hard stainless-steel wire (*Figure 8.39A–D*):

   A. Casts on the articulator.

   B. Upper labial arch with U-loops opposite canine teeth. Wire work for labial pads. This can be made in one piece but it is quicker and easier to use three pieces of wire for this part.

All the wires are attached to the casts with hard wax at points which will not subsequently interfere

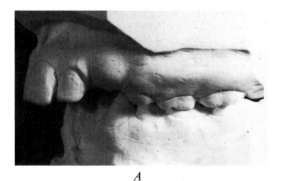

A

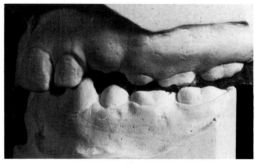

B

Figure 8.38 Construction of the function regulator. Taking the bite; *A*, postnormal occlusion; *B*, the mandible is brought forward and the teeth brought together into contact

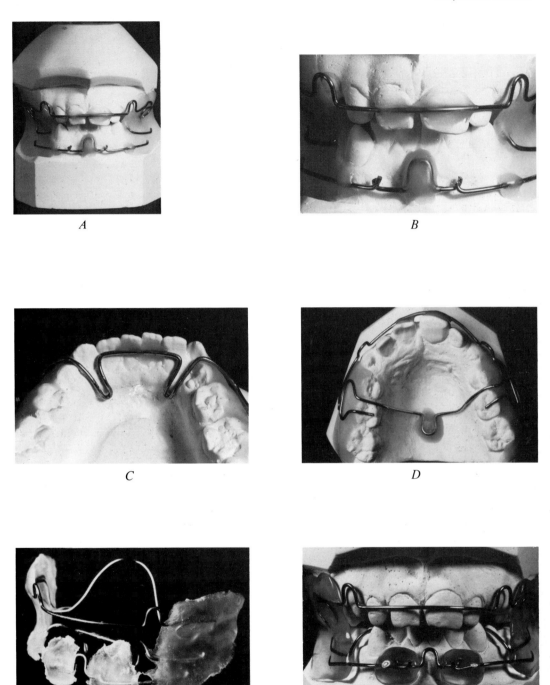

Figure 8.39 Construction of the wire assembly of the function corrector; *A*, the casts are placed on an articulator, the buccal segments are covered with a layer of wax, and the wire parts are formed; *B*, the upper and lower labial bows; *C*, the lower lingual arch with loops; *D*, the upper labial bow and the palatal arch, with central loop and occlusal rests; *E*, the complete appliance with the resin polymerised; *F–H*, the appliance trimmed, polished and replaced upon the dental casts

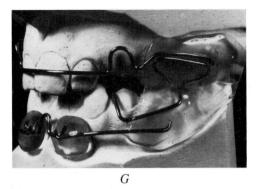

G

H

Figure 8.39 continued

with the application of the cold curing resin. All the tag ends of the wires are brought buccally for anchorage in the buccal shields.

C. It is recommended by Fränkel that the lower lingual arch be made in 0.9 mm soft wire. It has been found in practice that hard wire may be used and that arches made of hard wire do not become distorted or broken.

D. Palatal arch with central U-loop. This arch must stand clear of the palate by 1–2 mm and pass buccally between the occlusal surfaces of the cheek teeth. The ends of the archwire are formed into loops for anchorage in the buccal shields and then brought towards the midline to make rests lying on the occlusal surfaces of the upper second deciduous molars. If these teeth are not present the rests should lie upon the first permanent molars.

4. The articulator is closed and the buccal wax padding made good at the line of the occlusion. A separating medium is applied to the plaster where the labial pads are to be constructed.

5. Cold curing clear acrylic material is used to build up the buccal wings and labial pads.

6. Curing of the resin may be accelerated by the use of a hydraulic pressure flask filled with lukewarm water. To get the appliance into the flask, the casts are removed together from the articulator and their bases cut down as much as necessary by means of a model grinder.

Using a hydraulic flask the resin sets rapidly, is free of porosity and the heat involved is not enough to soften the wax and disturb the relative positions of the casts (*Figure 8.39E*).

7. When the resin has set all the wax is removed from the casts with hot water.

8. The appliance is trimmed and polished (*Figure 8.39F–H*)

9. An F.R.3 appliance is shown in *Figure 8.40*.

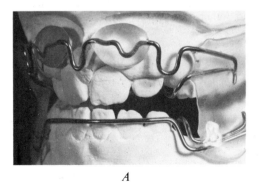

A

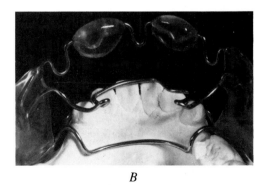

B

Figure 8.40 The F.R.3 appliance; *A*, the labial pads are lying under the upper lip and a labial bow lies against the lower incisors; *B*, note that the lower lingual arch stands away from the lower incisors and alveolar process. There is an upper lingual arch which touches the upper incisors

Management of the appliance

When the appliance is fitted the patient will be able to say at once whether there are any spots of discomfort or excessive pressure on teeth or soft tissues. Any such defects must be removed by adjusting the wire or easing the acrylic material away from the labial mucosa. Pressure points under the screens or pads show as areas of blanching visible through the clear resin. The labial pads will, of course, lie against the alveolar mucosa when the appliance is first fitted and it is necessary to trim away an even thickness of from 1 mm to 2 mm from the alveolar surface of the pads. The depth to which the pads project into the labial sulcus must be carefully watched and, if there is any irritation of the mobile mucosa, the pads should be trimmed back at the offending spot and the trimmed surface polished.

Most patients will be able to wear the appliance full-time from the first visit and to carry on a normal daily routine, apart from eating, with the appliance in place.

A patient who is self-conscious may for an initial period of a fortnight wear the appliance only on coming home from school and at night. Thereafter it must be worn at all times except when eating. Very little maintenance or adjustment of the appliance is required apart from repair of accidental damage.

Indications for the use of the function corrector

The following set of case reports is the material of an investigation into indications for the use of functional correctors (Adams, 1969), published in the *Transactions of the European Orthodontic Society* for that year and reproduced by permission. The material has been grouped in the following way:

1. Postnormal occlusion (16 cases).
2. Prenormal occlusion (2 cases).
3. Anterior open bite (1 case).

The postnormal occlusions treated were all of the Class II division 1 type and, as will be recognized, this includes a great many variations. Further classification of this group of 16 cases was carried out as follows.

Subdivisions of Class II division 1 malocclusion

1. Slight uncomplicated (2 cases).
2. Severe uncomplicated (5 cases).
3. With thumb sucking (4 cases).
4. With crowding (5 cases).
5. With early loss of deciduous teeth (3 cases).

Some cases came into more than one group and were therefore considered under more than one heading.

The postnormal occlusions and the open bite cases were treated with the F.R.1 type of appliance and the prenormal occlusions with the F.R.3. The results were as follows:

Postnormal occlusion
Good result   4 cases
No improvement   12 cases
Open bite
Good result   1 case
Prenormal occlusion
Good result   2 cases

Before discussing these results it is necessary to examine in more detail a few of the cases that were successfully treated and what occurred in them.

Postnormal occlusion

The cases in question were:

1. A girl in whom a severe malocclusion existed from the time of eruption of the deciduous dentition until the problem was treated with the F.R.1 at age 10 (category 2).
2. Two boys in whom there was crowding of the dentition, early loss of deciduous teeth and a severe postnormal occlusion (categories 4 and 5).
3. A boy aged 3 years 2 months with a gross postnormal occlusion and with lip sucking habits. Otherwise there was adequate room in the dental arches (category 2).

Case reports

1. J. M. (*Figures 8.41–8.44*).

This patient attended aged 3 years 6 months with a history of lip sucking but not thumb sucking, although the appearance of the teeth strongly suggested a digit-sucking habit. The patient's mother was emphatic that any thumb sucking that took place was very occasional. The subsequent treatment result confirmed that the digit habit was of no importance in this case and the parent's assessment was absolutely correct.

Diagnosis

A marked discrepancy in facial proportions was found with postnormality of the mandible and although the lips were of adequate proportions the lower lip lay continuously under the upper incisors and on swallowing the lower lip contracted firmly against the tongue (*Figure 8.41A*).

A simple cephalometric analysis revealed that the SNA/B difference was high, 8°, lower incisors retroclined to 73° to mandibular plane, and the upper incisors proclined to 114.5° to the maxillary plane. There was a large overjet and incomplete, non-increased overbite (*Figure 8.41B–D*).

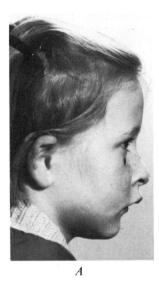

A

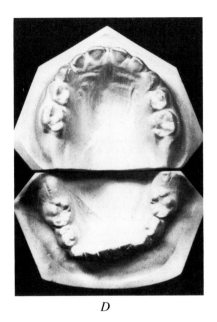

D

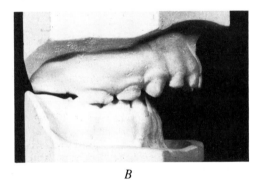

B

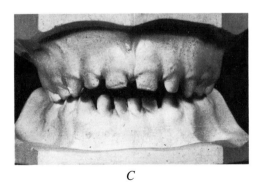

C

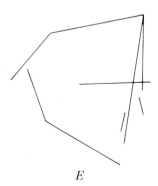

E

Figure 8.41 J.M. aged 3 years 6 months; *A*, profile; *B–D*, dental casts. Note that in occlusal view the lower incisors appear to be pushed lingually, especially on the left, and the upper incisors are forward on the right; *E*, tracing of cephalometric film

Treatment planning

The patient was so small and so young that no active treatment was initiated at this stage, but yearly visits were instituted to observe growth progress and record by casts and cephalometric films the changes that were taking place.

At the age of 7 years the occlusion, facial pattern and soft-tissue activities were just as they had always been, the only difference was that permanent lower incisors were up instead of deciduous ones (*Figure 8.42A* and *B*). At this stage it was felt that something must be done to mitigate the condition and an attempt was made to align the lower labial segment to a more forward position. The movement required being a simple proclination a removable appliance was used, but it was not possible to produce the tooth movement as planned; the teeth would not move but instead became loose and it was deemed wiser after a short time not to continue with this line of treatment.

Subsequently an Andresen appliance was placed for a period of 9 months at the age of 8 years, but as this treatment produced not the slightest change in the occlusion the appliance was abandoned. An oral screen was also used for a short time but was also withdrawn quite soon.

Finally, it was decided that the function corrector might help the patient and at the age of 10 years the child was put on to function regulator treatment and within a few weeks improvements in the occlusal relationships began to take place. At the end of 14 months, both upper and lower dental arch arrangement was excellent and incisor relationship was nearly normal, mainly due to proclination of the lower incisors, although the upper incisors had retroclined to some degree (*Figure 8.43A* and *B*).

The Fränkel appliance was continued for a further 7 months, at the end of which time no further improvement in occlusal relationship had taken place and, as the molar relation was still postnormal, treatment was changed to the use of an Andresen appliance which produced some further occlusal improvement. The Andresen appliance was being worn until the age of 12 years 9 months (*Figure 8.44A–E*).

Assessment of the result

There is no doubt that in this case a rapid and dramatic improvement was made in the occlusion for this patient, although the appearance of the patient in profile does not appear greatly different before and after treatment as regards the relative prognathism of the upper and lower dental bases. The angle ANB at the end of treatment was 6°, a little less than the original 8° when the patient was first seen and 1° less than the 7° at the beginning of treatment. The mandible appears to have swung a little downwards and forwards during the time the patient has been under supervision and this may account for the change in ANB. The change in this angle of 2° appears to be due to an increase in the angle SNB of 2°, although the intermediate reduction in ANB of 1° seems to be due to a reduction in SNA of that amount.

The strong impression remains that the improvements that are to be seen in the occlusion are not due to changes in the basic face shape but to changes in the arrangement of the teeth within the the facial outlines. During the course of treatment the lower incisors have become proclined from 72.5° to the mandibular plane to 92.5°, a change of 20°, and the upper incisors have been retroclined by 6° to the maxillary plane. The changes in the molar region have been noticeable but by no means as striking. The patient's ability to keep a normal lip position and activity has been greatly improved and will be

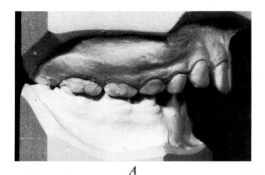

A

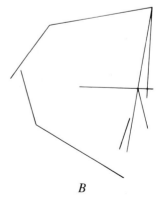

B

Figure 8.42 J.M. aged 8 years 8 months; *A*, dental casts; *B*, cephalometric tracing

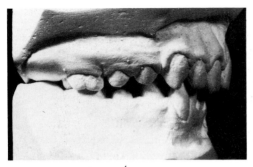

A

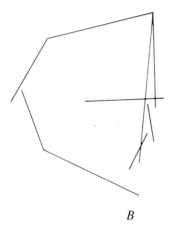

B

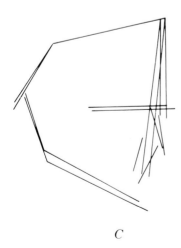

C

Figure 8.43 J.M. aged 11 years 2 months; *A*, dental casts, right view; *B*, tracing at 11 years 2 months; (*C*), superimposition of tracings at 8 years 8 months and 11 years 2 months

an important factor in the ultimate stability of the new occlusal relationship.

2. G. J. (*Figures 8.45–8.47*).

Diagnosis

This patient, a boy aged 8 years 8 months, attended showing a severe degree of postnormality of dental bases and a similar discrepancy in the occlusion aggravated by early loss of deciduous teeth and closure of spaces for the unerupted premolar teeth. In this case there was no recorded anomaly of function of the orofacial musculature apart from a posture of the lower lip below the upper incisors. It was envisaged from the outset that teeth should be removed as part of treatment eventually to deal with the problem of crowding (*Figure 8.45*).

Treatment

A Fränkel 1 appliance was used in view of the severity of the overjet and overbite in an attempt to produce some improvement pending the eruption of the permanent canine and premolar teeth.

Changes for the better began to take place within a few weeks and by the time 8 months had passed there was a very marked improvement (*Figure 8.46*). The appliance was worn for a further year because improvement appeared to be continuing. The premolars were then beginning to erupt and after a further 6 months extraction of the upper first premolars was advised to allow the canine teeth to erupt (*Figure 8.47*).

Assessment

What were the changes that took place in this case? There is no doubt of the improvement that occurred in the incisor relationship and the tracings of the cephalometric films seem to show that the change is due to alteration in axial inclinations. It is impossible to say about which point the teeth inclined because the bone areas in which the teeth are supported have changed in position. It should, however, be noted that the relative positions of the anterior part of the jaws themselves as indicated by SNA and SNB remained the same. The relationship of the molar teeth on the two sides did not behave in the same way. On the right there was little if any change, while on the left a postnormal molar relationship of one unit improved to a half-unit postnormality. There was no obvious explanation as to how this had come about.

Prognosis

It was noted in this case that there was no anomaly of function apart from a resting of the lower lip below the upper incisors, a condition which no longer obtains as the new incisor relationship now

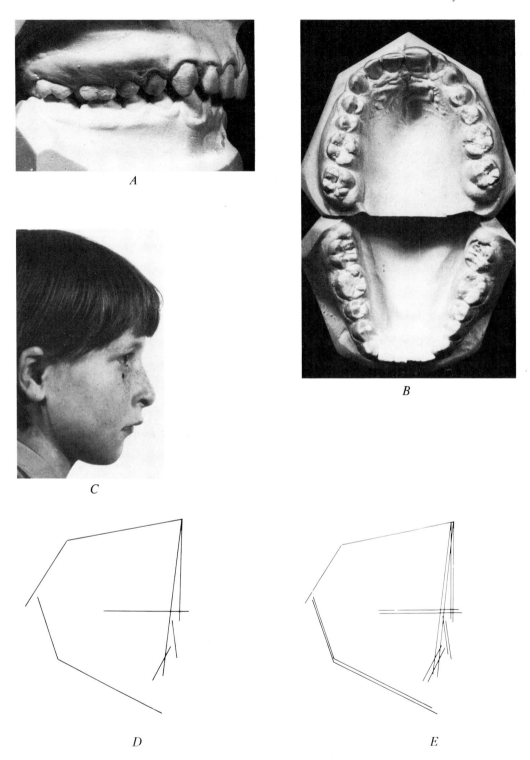

Figure 8.44 J.M. aged 12 years 4 months; *A* and *B*, dental casts, right and occlusal views. Note in occlusal view the symmetrical and well-arranged arches; *C*, profile. Compare with *Figure 8.42*; *D*, tracing at 12 years 4 months; *E*, superimposition of tracings at 11 years 2 months and 12 years 4 months

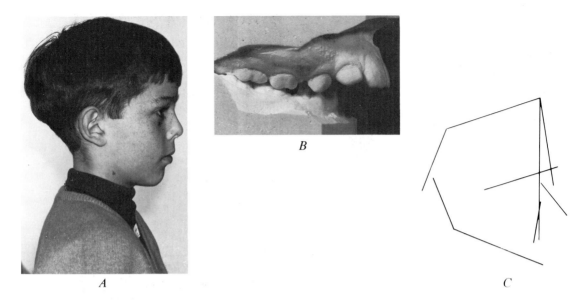

Figure 8.45 G.J. aged 8 years 11 months; *A*, profile; *B*, casts, right lateral view; *C*, tracing of cephalometric film

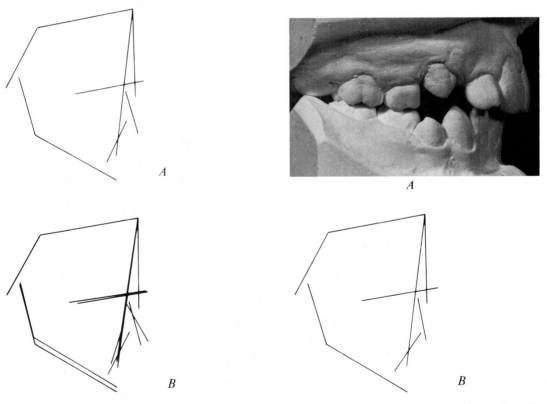

Figure 8.46 G.J; *A*, tracing at age 9 years 7 months; *B*, tracing at 8 years 11 months and 9 years 7 months superimposed. Upper incisors are retroclined, lower incisors are proclined

Figure 8.47 G.J. *A*, dental casts at age 10 years 7 months; *B*, tracing at 10 years 7 months

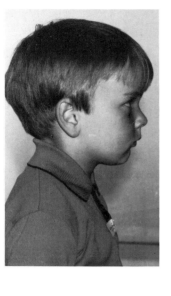

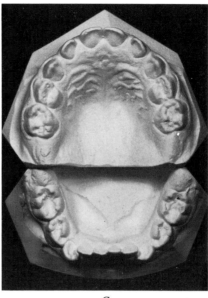

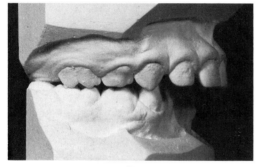

A

C

B

Figure 8.48 W.McK. aged 3 years; *A*, profile; *B* and *C*, dental casts, right and occlusal views

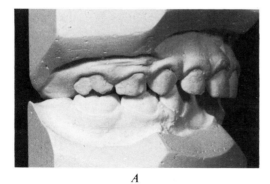

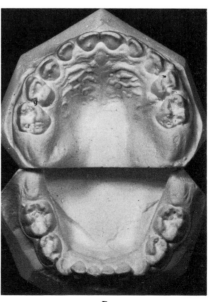

A

B

Figure 8.49 W.McK. aged 4 years 3 months; *A* and *B*, dental casts, right and occlusal views. Note slight improvement in arrangement of lower incisors

permits correct lip posture at rest. In these circumstances conditions are favourable for stability of the new incisor relationship. The crowding of the dental arches is to be treated by removal of first premolars and the final occlusal relationship of the buccal segments has yet to be worked out.

3. W. McK. (*Figures 8.48, 8.49*).

Diagnosis

This boy, aged 3 years, was brought for advice because of an open bite condition and marked retrognathism. On examination the patient was found to have a postnormal dental base relation, incompetent lips, and a marked lower lip-sucking/tongue-thrusting oral activity. The occlusion was markedly postnormal and there was a considerable overbite. There was no thumb sucking (*Figure 8.48*).

Treatment

The patient was given an F.R.1 appliance and took to it at once and has worn the appliance without any difficulty for 1 year 3 months.

There was considerable improvement in the occlusion in that time and the patient is to continue to wear the appliance as long as improvements continue to take place (*Figure 8.49*). The author is not sure that it would be wise simply to continue to use the appliance indefinitely and if a static condition is reached a resting period from treatment should be allowed, in all probability during the eruption of the permanent dentition, and when these teeth are erupted the whole problem should be reviewed in the light of the circumstances then found.

Prenormal occlusion

Case reports

1. T.K. (*Figures 8.50 and 8.51*).

Diagnosis

This patient, aged 9 years, had a severe Class III malocclusion due in part to a mesial displacement of the mandible on closing from the position of rest to the centric occlusal position, and also to a basic discrepancy in facial proportions in the direction of a mandibular prognathism. The large degree of overlap of the incisors and the break-up of the occlusal line in the buccal segments suggest that there is some overclosure in this case, a condition that goes with premature contact, muscle spasm, failure of eruption of teeth in the buccal segments, and reduction of the normal maxillo-mandibular vertical height dimension (*Figure 8.50*).

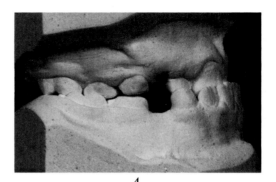

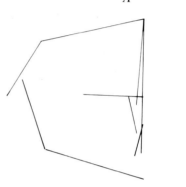

Figure 8.50 T.K. aged 9 years; *A*, dental casts, right view; *B*, tracing of headfilm

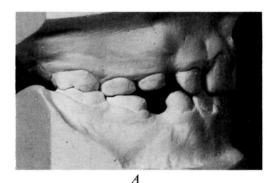

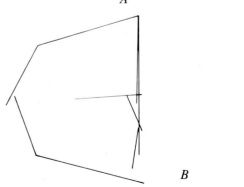

Figure 8.51 T.K. aged 9 years 7 months; *A*, dental casts; *B*, cephalometric tracing

Treatment

The condition was treated with an F.R.3 appliance and after a period of 4 months from the time the appliance was fitted a great improvement in the occlusion had taken place; so much so that correct incisor relationship had been produced. The appliance was worn for a further 8 months because the degree of overbite of the incisors was not judged to be sufficient to ensure stability. After a total period of 12 months the appliance was withdrawn and the second cephalometric film was taken 2 months later (*Figure 8.51*).

An examination of the dental casts and the cephalometric tracings showed that the changes that had taken place were due to a repositioning of the mandible distally and to a slight proclination of the upper incisor teeth. The maxillomandibular separation also appears to have increased considerably, although the angular position of the mandibular body has not appreciably changed.

2. A second case of prenormal occlusion was also treated with the F.R.3 appliance and it is interesting to note that there were strong similarities in the general appearance of the occlusion and also in the reaction to treatment. It seemed that in both cases there was an element of displacement so that it is impossible to say from the evidence of these cases what is the effect of the appliance on true Class III malocclusion, that is to say, mandibular prognathism uncomplicated by any mesial displacement.

Anterior open bite

Case report

M. B. (*Figures 8.52–8.54*).

Diagnosis

This boy was brought for advice at the age of 6 years with a marked open bite, a tongue thrust and lip contraction on swallowing and speech (*Figure 8.52*).

It was felt that little could be accomplished by any form of active treatment in this case and the patient was dismissed for a period of 3 years, returning at the age of 9 years 3 months (*Figure 8.53*).

The permanent incisors had erupted but the open bite condition remained much as it had been when the patient first attended. The patient was dismissed for a further year after which, at the age of 10 years 3 months, an F.R.1 appliance was fitted and worn for a period of 11 months. During this time a considerable improvement in the open bite condition occurred, after which the appliance was left out (*Figure 8.54*).

A record of this patient taken 7 months later showed no further change in the overbite relationship. It appeared reasonable to conclude that it is

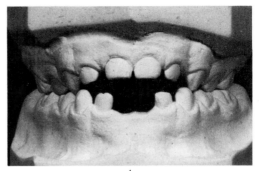

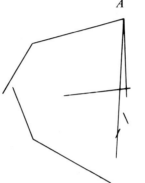

Figure 8.52 M.B. aged 5 years 9 months; *A*, dental casts; *B*, cephalometric tracing

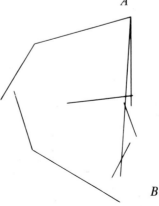

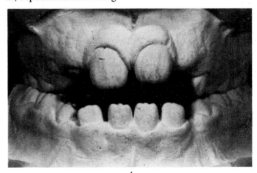

Figure 8.53 M.B. aged 9 years 3 months; *A*, dental casts; *B*, cephalometric tracing

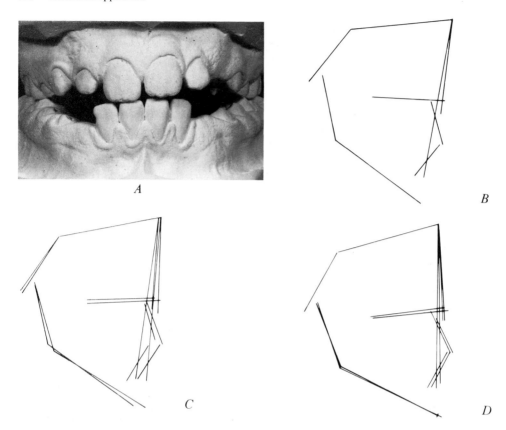

Figure 8.54 M.B. aged 11 years; *A*, dental casts; *B*, cephalometric tracing; *C*, superimposed tracings at 9 years 3 months and 11 years; *D*, superimposed tracings at 11 years and 11 years 7 months

very likely that the improvement in the overbite relationship was caused by the use of the appliance rather than that the change was taking place naturally during the time the appliance was being worn.

It is interesting to note that during the time when the appliance was being worn there has been, apparently, a forward and upward developmental change in the outline of the mandible. It is tempting to conclude that this must account for the improvement in the overbite. A study of the final stage of 7 months over which records were taken shows that the change in mandibular positioning has continued, although the incisor relationship has not continued to improve.

The remaining successful cases

The other cases in which good results were obtained showed many of the features which have been described in these four subjects. A degree of open bite was often present, possibly due to tongue and

lip activities, occlusal relationship markedly disturbed mesially or distally, and discrepancies in incisor relationships usually severe postnormally or prenormally. In all the cases that have been examined the changes that have been found to take place appeared to be limited to the dentoalveolar structures. In no case could it be said there was any evidence to suggest that basic jaw relationship had changed in any marked degree. This is surprising in view of the large changes in occlusal relationships, especially in the incisor region, that were observed clinically. Closer examination by means of cephalometric films only revealed changes in tooth inclinations.

Changes in skull base angle and in mandibular posture within the craniofacial complex were found but these changes were not reflected in any change in the measurements by which relationship between upper and lower dental bases is usually judged. These observations support the idea that the Fränkel appliance acts by mediating the apposition of bone on surfaces rather than by promoting

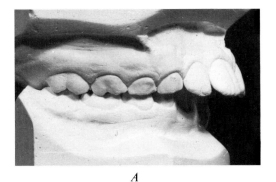

A

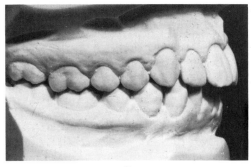

B

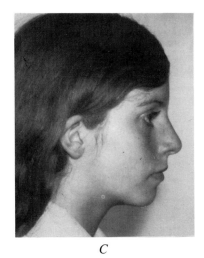

C

Figure 8.55 Postnormal occlusion and the functional regulator. This patient's treatment was started at age 10 years in the early stages of the changeover to the permanent dentition in the buccal segments. The final result fulfilled the highest expectations as treatment by any other means was not compatible with the patient's stage career; *A*, at age 10 before treatment; *B*, final record casts age 15; *C*, profile at age 15

change in the relationship of the two parts of the masticatory face as a whole.

Figure 8.55 shows a patient of 9.5 years in the mixed dentition. There is a well-marked Class II division 1 malocclusion with increased overjet and overbite but no spacing in the anterior teeth. It was decided in this case to treat with a functional regulator and this proved most successful producing, in the end, normal occlusion with improvement of overbite and overjet. It can be seen that the patient has a slightly postnormal dental base relationship but competent lip posture.

The cases that failed

What can be said about the cases that did not improve with the use of the function corrector?

The first thing is that in the material available for this investigation the cases that failed were all in the Class II division 1 group. The subjects did not differ greatly from those in whom the treatment was a success, with one important exception, and this is the group of three subjects in whom there was a thumb-sucking habit.

To some extent it appeared that the influence of the thumb did not counteract the effect of the appliance as such, but rather because the appliance interfered with the activity of the thumb, which was one of the aims of treatment, in the cases in question it was not the thumb which gave way but the appliance.

In one case in which the parent was more than usually active and interested in the progress of treatment it was stated that the appliance was felt to be an affront to the thumb-sucking activity and the thumb was greatly preferred to the appliance. In the other thumb-sucking cases no effect was produced by the appliance at all and, although the day-to-day use of the appliance was not reported and documented, it seemed very likely that the appliances were not worn.

As regards the other four categories, these may be divided into those in whom there was non-cooperation in wearing the appliance, although the malocclusions seemed basically amenable to treatment by the system, and those in whom there was cooperation. In the first of these groups of cases appliances were left out, lost and broken so that the time during which the appliances were in position must have been very small. It seemed clear that in some of these cases the fault did not lie entirely with the patient. It was found that the appliance was sometimes not comfortable to wear because it was unstable and the screens did not, in consequence, lie in the proper positions or stood too far out from the alveolar process or the tooth crowns. Sometimes the mandible had been brought too far forwards, so producing discomfort and difficulty in speech and causing the appliance to tilt and hold the lips in a completely wrong position.

In the remaining cases, as far as could be ascertained, there was good cooperation and parental interest and anxiety to achieve a good result.

Even so, the results were disappointing, with small changes only or no change at all after wearing the appliances. Two further aspects of these cases in which there was cooperation appeared to be of significance, one of which was that there was a well-defined dental base discrepancy and usually associated with this was the fact that there was no anomaly of tongue or lip activity.

Conclusions

As more clinical experience has been gained with these appliances, the results of cephalometric investigations into their effects in larger groups of subjects have become available.

McNamara *et al.* (1985) have recorded the effects of function regulators in treating 99 subjects with Class II division 1 malocclusion. These authors preferred a palatal wire behind the upper incisors in the function regulator in the treatment of Class II division 1. Kerr and TenHave (1988) investigated the effects in treating 30 subjects with Class III malocclusion.

The results from these two studies have been used to compare the effects of the F.R.2 with those of the F.R.3 and, in particular, to ascertain whether there were any changes in the configuration of the basic shape of the face that might be attributable to the appliance treatment. Attention was, therefore, directed particularly to possible changes in the dental bases.

The mean ages of the two groups were 10.2 years for the Class II cases and 10.5 for the Class III. The results of this comparison indicated that the non-dental changes produced by both types of appliances were on the mandible and that the angle SNA showed a slight annual mean reduction in the Class II division 1 group. This group also showed a greater annual mean increase in mandibular length of 1.2 mm over the treatment period than did the

control group, a normative sample drawn from the University of Michigan Growth Study. This increase was largely due to an increase in mandibular ramus height. The restraint in point A and the advancement of point B produced an annual mean decrease of 0.9 mm in angle ANB.

The Class III group showed a reduction in the angle SNB which appeared to be accounted for by a spatial change in mandibular position downwards and backwards. Enlow's mandibular skeletal distance measured along a line parallel to the functional occlusal plane to a defined posterior limit (Enlow *et al.*, 1969; Riolo *et al.*, 1974) showed a reduction and an increase in cranial base angle helped to relocate the mandibular condyle further posteriorly.

The superimposed tracings of the two malocclusion groups can be seen in *Figure 8.56*. These tracings demonstrate the difference between the two facial types before treatment and the tendency for both groups to some rapprochement at the end of active treatment.

Although the long-term effects of these appliances have yet to be fully assessed, there is

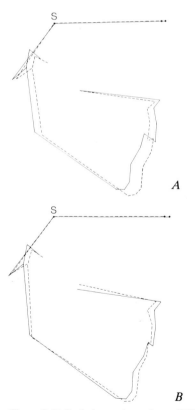

Figure 8.56 Cephalometric tracings of F.R.2 and F.R.3. Group means superimposed on SN registered at S; *A*, before treatment; *B*, after treatment. F.R.2, solid line; F.R.3, broken line

evidence from these studies to support the concept that function regulators can exert some influence on mandibular growth and posture. From the point of view of the clinical orthodontist, the use of functional appliances will raise in his mind the question of whether the treatments he undertakes will improve the appearance of the patient's face as well as the arrangements of the patient's teeth. In patients who have markedly discrepant facial profiles there are inevitable limitations on the improvements that can be made in appearance and masticatory function by readjustments in the positions of the teeth alone. It is, therefore, worth knowing whether changes in the overall relationships of the facial profile, including changes in the anteroposterior relationship of the basic elements of the face, the mandible and maxilla, can be effected by orthopaedic means.

It is a common observation that many patients who have severe Class III malocclusions are more concerned with the appearance of their chins than the functionally and aesthetically disadvantageous appearance and relationship of their incisor teeth and for that reason will agree to surgical treatment.

The orthodontist is striving to produce results within the limitations imposed by the basic shape of the face and if it can be shown that facial shape can be influenced by functional means, the way is open for the treatment of severe malocclusions by means that stop short of surgical interference with the basic supporting structures of the dentition.

Two further examples of treatment of prenormal occlusion are shown in *Figures 8.57* and *8.58*. D.McA. was a boy of 8 years 6 months and S.E. a girl of 8 years 7 months on presentation. Both had severe Class III malocclusions with ANB discrepancies of $-2°$ and $-3°$ respectively. In both cases the overbite was deep and the upper incisors were already proclined with respect to the maxillary plane so that simple proclination of these teeth alone was contraindicated.

The superimposed before-and-after tracings show the treatment effects of the F.R.3 to be similar in the two cases, namely an increase in angle ANB, $+3°$ and $+2°$ respectively, facilitated by some opening of the cranial base angle and a downwards and backwards rotation of the mandible. The upper incisors were minimally proclined in both cases, $4°$, and the lower incisors retroclined $4°$ and $7°$ respectively.

1. What should the Fränkel appliance be used for?
2. In what kind of cases may success be hoped for?
3. What is one entitled to expect from the appliance if properly used?

1. The Fränkel appliance has been shown to produce improvement of the occlusion in Class II and Class III malocclusions and in open bite so that any cases of these types may be considered for treatment by the function corrector. It has not been the authors' experience that the appliance helps the condition of crowding as such, although in some of the successfully treated Class II division 1 cases crowding was present. The need to extract teeth for the relief of crowding remained and this need was foreseen, although the malocclusion as a whole improved.

2. The appliance has been found to work successfully in cases in which there is a severe discrepancy of dental base and occlusal relationship, in which there is a severe anomaly of function of the tongue and lips, and in which there have been crowding and early loss of deciduous teeth. In cases in the present series in which there was a thumb-sucking habit no improvement was produced. This may be an indication for caution in the use of the appliance in such cases.

3. What may one expect from the use of the appliance?
(a) It is the authors' experience that, if the appliance is going to work, changes will take place rapidly. If this does not occur, it is likely that the appliance is not going to be successful and after a period of about 4 months the diagnosis and treatment plan should be carefully reconsidered.
(b) The changes that take place are mainly to be seen in the anterior teeth and are produced by changes in axial inclination of the teeth.
(c) Changes in the anteroposterior occlusion of the teeth in the buccal segments will be small and it is the authors' practice to produce such changes by other means than the function corrector.
(d) Changes in the relationship of the teeth appear to be produced by rearrangement of the dento-alveolar structures and not by changes in the basal relationships of the jaws.
(e) The appliance seems to have a valuable part to play in certain cases in the mixed dentition stage of development when the fitting of precisely constructed removable or fixed appliances may be disturbed by the loss of deciduous teeth.
(f) The appliance can be used in young subjects and, when severe malocclusions are present, a start can be given to improvement of occlusal relationship.
(g) The relationship between the orthodontist and the patient is important in eliciting cooperation. It is important that the patient should accept the appliance and virtually forget that it is being worn.

The function corrector is a most useful appliance in the treatment of a proportion of cases of certain types. The number of cases included in the present investigation is very small, so small as to make it perhaps unwise to try to draw any general conclusions from them. A careful, accurate and dispassionate appraisal of the effects of treatment in even a small number of cases can be shown to be informative, revealing and helpful in the planning of future applications of the system.

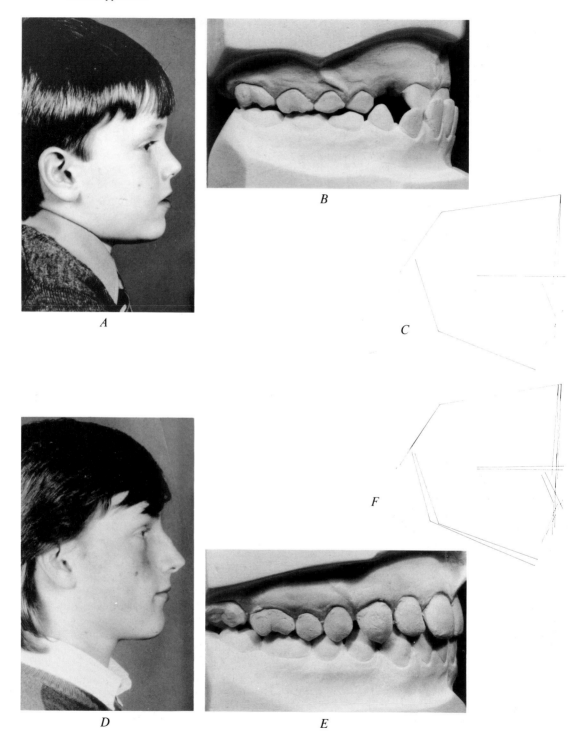

Figure 8.57 D.McA.; *A–C*, profile photograph, cephalometric tracing and study models before treatment, age 8 years 6 months; *D* and *E*, profile photograph and study models at 15 years 3 months, some years after active treatment; *F*, cephalometric tracings before and after F.R.3 treatment, superimposed on SN registered at S (8 years 6 months/9 years 7 months)

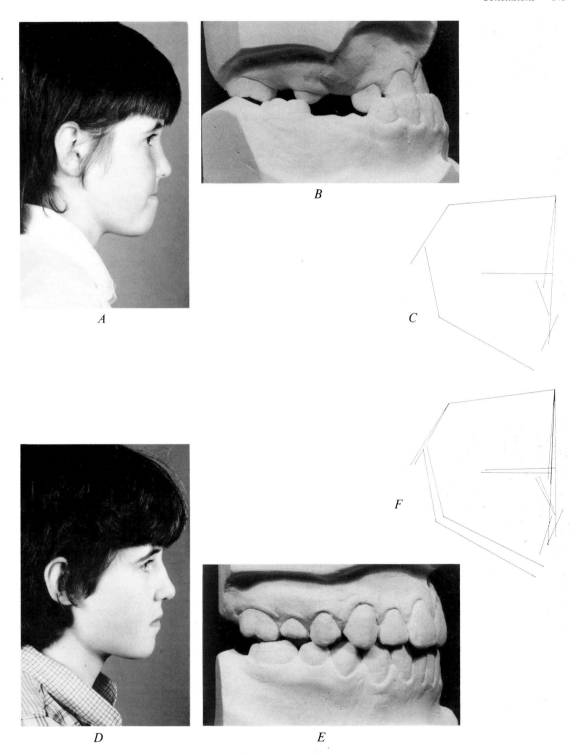

Figure 8.58 S.E.; *A–C*, profile photograph, cephalometric tracing and study models before treatment, age 8 years 7 months; *D* and *E*, profile photograph and study models at 13 years 6 months, some years after active treatment; *F*, cephalometric tracings before and after F.R.3 treatment, superimposed on SN registered at S (8 years 7 months/10 years)

The way forward with functional appliances

In this chapter, attention has been given to two of the best known types of functional appliances which operate in basically different ways, the Andresen appliance and the Fränkel appliance. These appliances have been widely used for many years in Europe and are being increasingly used in the United States of America and in Canada. They have been the subjects of hypotheses, investigation, experimentation and modification.

Functional appliances have their proponents and their opponents but the advantages of treatment of major malocclusions by what might be considered comparatively non-invasive means are too great for functional treatment methods to be left out of the available schemes of management of malocclusion.

There are many mixtures of the principles of action of functional appliances in the various apparatuses that are available today, and each mixture strives for greater efficacy in producing better and more permanent results. It may be, indeed, that as in medicine, in a combination of agents, adjuvant effects occur and the whole effect may be greater than the sum of the individual parts.

In assessing how a functional appliance is working it is well, therefore, to think of where the influences are coming from, the masticatory muscles, the facial and lingual muscles, the placing of the mandible out of its usual relationship with the maxilla, the influences of pressure elements embodied in the appliance.

In determining the effects produced by any functional system of treatment, it is necessary to evaluate the changes produced in tooth position within the jaws, in the shape, size and relationship of the jaws and in the muscular and other tissues investing and connected to the jaws. It is also above all necessary to discount the changes that must be expected in growth during the period when treatment was being done.

The Harvold Andresen appliance

An evaluation has been done by Harvold and Vargervik (1971) of a new kind of Andresen appliance which differs from the pattern that has been widely used in the past (*Figure 8.59*).

The Andresen appliance advocated by Harvold (1974) is used in the early mixed and mixed dentition. The bite is taken in a very open position and is supported on the anterior teeth which are at the same time left free to incline. The upper molar teeth are propped on a plane to prevent eruption and the lower molars are encouraged to erupt further. The hypothesis underlying these arrangements is that correction of the occlusal relationship in Class II division 1 malocclusion is dependent less on changes in jaw relationship or in anteroposterior tooth position than on eruption of the lower molar teeth and that this is what should be aimed at through treatment with this functional appliance.

Other improvements in the orofacial complex which are part of the treatment plan by this method include the correction of incisor inclinations, overjet and overbite and strengthening and adjusting muscle activity to maintain the new tooth arrangements.

It is also thought that these improvements will lead to improvements in nasal respiration.

Other functional appliances

Other functional appliance systems combine, in varying degree, means to posture the mandible, screen the dentition from the pressures of tongue and lips, exert individual pressures on teeth or groups of teeth, and invoke the aid of traction using the head and neck as a base for anchorage.

One such system has been put forward by Clark (1982) which invokes all these factors in a single appliance system.

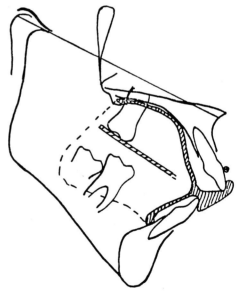

Figure 8.59 This diagram shows the principal features of the Andresen appliance as modified by Harvold (1974). The working bite is taken fairly widely open, the appliance cut away from the anterior teeth and from their bony support so that the teeth can incline freely. There is an upper labial bow which can be activated to produce retroclination of the upper incisors. The occlusion is propped mainly on the incisal edges of the anterior teeth and on the upper molars, which rest on platforms to prevent their eruption or 'extrusion' as it is referred to. The lower molars are free to erupt

Functional appliance treatment is at the very foundation of orthodontics or, as it is sometimes termed, dentofacial orthopaedics. Perhaps the most important aspect of the functional approach to treatment is that treatment regimens which take control of the occlusion and place the teeth and dental arches in predetermined positions must, sooner or later, let go. The functional forces of the occlusion then take over and finally determine where everything shall come to rest.

It is possible that treatment changes produced by functional means may require little settling down after treatment is completed and the result may be nearer to the final positions of the teeth under the influence of natural forces than if that result were obtained by more mechanical means.

Chapter 9

Patient and appliance management

Introduction

Removable appliances offer a very simple means for the management of certain kinds of tooth irregularities and for some stages in more elaborate treatment problems. The advantages of removable appliances soon become apparent to the user in such circumstances.

The fact that these appliances are removable ensures that there is no impediment to the maintenance of a high level of oral hygiene and in the event of discomfort or breakage, an appliance can be removed to avoid damage to the teeth and oral tissues. Other dental procedures such as preventive and restorative treatments can proceed without hindrance during the course of removable appliance therapy. As the appliances are constructed on plaster casts and adjustments made outside the mouth, the amount of chairside time necessary for their management and inconvenience to the patient are reduced. Removable appliances provide considerably more anchorage than fixed appliances as a consequence of mucosal coverage by the baseplates and the palatal vault is particularly helpful in resisting anchorage slip during distal movement of upper teeth.

Removable appliances are very much under the control of the patient and it is important that the patient is in the confidence of the operator and plays his part by cooperating in wearing his appliances, by keeping them and his own mouth clean, by handling appliances carefully when inserting and removing them and by refraining from eating foodstuffs of a hard or adhesive nature such as would damage appliances. It is necessary to consider carefully whether it is possible to treat a patient with any kind of orthodontic appliance if he will not cooperate. A patient who is only compliant, who agrees under persuasion or duress to have treatment cannot be treated as satisfactorily, if he can even be treated at all, as a patient who wishes to have treatment, understands what is being done and cooperates willingly and actively in the treatment procedures.

After a treatment plan and prognosis have been explained to the parent and agreement reached on these matters, a frank discussion with the patient, without the presence of the parent, is the best way of assessing the patient's interest, understanding and wish to cooperate in the treatment of his problem.

Orthodontic treatment lies between the orthodontist, the patient and the appliance. In the last resort, there is little the parent can do if the patient avails himself of every opportunity to put aside or damage his orthodontic appliance when at school, at play or when out of the parent's sight. The patient and the orthodontist must be in total rapport; the parent can only tell the orthodontist anything he notices going on, should all not be well, and the patient is primarily in control.

A number of studies have been carried out in attempts to assess the overall usefulness of removable and other appliances in orthodontic treatment from the point of view of what proportion of patients discontinued treatment and at what age and what was the breakage rate for removable appliances (Haynes, 1982; Kerr, 1984; Woollass et al., 1988). While such studies may have some value, they are of little relevance if isolated from similar studies concerning fixed appliances which by their nature have many more separate parts and are as likely or more likely to suffer damage at the hands of uncooperative patients and lead to abandonment of treatment.

Skilful users of removable appliances will have less trouble with broken appliances than maladroit operators and will be well able to assess and engender cooperation in patients who will like their orthodontists and wish to have their treatments successfully completed as soon as possible.

With these basic principles in mind, the management of removable appliances can be considered under the following headings.

Issuing the appliance

A removable appliance should be placed within two weeks of taking the impression so as to minimize the possiblility of tooth movements causing the appliance not to fit properly. If a tooth or a number of teeth are to be removed as part of treatment, extraction should be delayed, unless completely unavoidable, until the appliance is constructed and placed. To ensure the best possible fit of a removable appliance in the young, developing dentition an appliance should be placed within a few days of taking the impression. If teeth have just been extracted, even a few day's delay in placing an appliance will cause an unacceptable lack of fit.

Appliances should be delivered to the clinic on the casts on which they were constructed so that the prescription can be checked and the design and fit of clasps and springs examined. Prior to placing the appliance in the mouth, the clinician should ensure that there are no minute pimples due to blow holes in the plaster cast that could irritate the mucosa and that the free edges, distal edge in an upper appliance and lower edge in a lower appliance, are rounded and smoothed.

Clasps should fit the teeth accurately and the arrowheads should lie against the spots on the teeth where the mesial and distal undercuts occur. Clasps need not actually grasp the teeth at this stage; the required retention of the appliance is effected by adjusting the clasps to the correct degree of tension. In no sense are clasps fitted when an appliance is placed. If clasps do not fit, the fault lies at some stage in the construction of the appliance and an appliance with clasps that do not fit properly should be rejected and a new start made (*see* Appendix B).

Bite-planes should be checked for height, width, anteroposterior depth and conformity to the teeth in the opposing arch biting on them, having regard to the purpose for which the bite-plane is being used.

An anterior bite-plane should be wide enough to allow the lower labial segment from canine to canine to make contact and deep enough anteroposteriorly to ensure that the lower labial segment cannot bite behind the back edge of the plane as may occur if there is a large overjet. In cases of a very deep overbite an anterior bite-plane may need to be built up in stages over a period of time using cold curing acrylic until sufficient bite opening is achieved.

Where posterior bite-planes are used to prop the bite open temporarily to permit proclination of upper incisors, the planes should be only deep enough to eliminate occlusal interference and permit proclination of the teeth. Such planes should be adjusted, using articulating paper, to balance the occlusal contact on both sides.

In adjusting both anterior and posterior bite-planes, bulk should be reduced to the necessary minimum as this will render the appliance more comfortable to wear and ensure good cooperation. Any unnecessary intrusion on the space for the tongue, which may occur if an anterior bite-plane comes too far distally or should posterior bite-planes be too wide, interferes with speech and embarrasses the patient. A quite small adjustment of a bite-plane can give just a little more space and cheer up a child who may be experiencing difficulty with a new appliance.

If tooth movement is ready to be started, springs may be adjusted at this time in most cases. If it is evident that the patient needs to have some time to get used to handling the appliance and inserting and removing it, the additional manoeuvre of getting springs into place may be left until the next visit. If extractions are needed, the adjustment of springs should be left until the teeth have been removed. In the meanwhile the patient will become accustomed to manipulating his appliance. The same applies to extra-oral components which can be added at a subsequent visit when the patient has acclimatized to the intra-oral parts.

Notwithstanding the phased management of appliance installation suggested, if a patient is intelligent, dexterous and motivated it is possible to complete all the stages of installation at a single visit. Patients vary enormously and some take to their appliances like ducks to water and others take more time to learn the ropes. It is a matter of making an accurate assessment of the patient's adaptability.

Once the clinician is satisfied that an appliance fits and is correctly adjusted, the next stage is to instruct the patient in the use and care of his appliance.

Instruction of the patient

It is one of the most important aspects of ensuring success with removable appliances that the patient and parent should be adequately counselled. Verbal advice may be reinforced with a fact sheet and a list of 'dos and don'ts'.

With the aid of a mirror the patient should be shown how to remove and insert the appliance, insisting that the appliance is not manoeuvred by the springs but by the bridges of the clasps. If the thumbs are placed on the occlusal surfaces of the upper buccal teeth, the first fingers can press downwards on the bridges of the clasps and the appliance is then grasped between the thumbs and first fingers by the bridges of the clasps. Merely to drag downwards on the clasps with the first fingers snaps the appliance off the dental arch into the mouth where it lies out of control.

Similarly, in the lower arch, the first fingers are placed on the occlusal surfaces of the buccal segments and the bridges of the clasps pressed up by the thumbs, the appliance being then grasped safely between first fingers and thumbs.

When inserting the appliance the patient is shown how to compress the springs so that they drop into position against the teeth to be moved and are not distorted.

The instruction to wear the appliance for 24 hours per day is then given, apart from removal for cleaning after meals. Well constructed appliances do not interfere with eating normal food or with speech, and patients should be assured that within a few days they will find no difficulty with eating and speaking.

A problem always arises with removable appliance-wearing in strenuous sports and contact games or in swimming and diving and in this connection it would be unwise to insist that there can be no relaxation of the rule that appliances can only be removed for cleaning. Common sense must prevail and if it is known that a patient is engaging in an activity in which an appliance could become dislodged and out of control, he should be instructed to carry a suitable box in which the appliance can be stored safely and returned to the mouth immediately after the activity is ceased.

Good patients are extremely resourceful and overcome seemingly impossible difficulties to ensure that their treatment is not interrupted while others will put aside appliances on the slightest pretext and perceive problems where they do not exist and always have a new excuse for every lapse.

A high standard of oral hygiene should be insisted on to avoid the possibility of enamel decalcification or gingival inflammation. Normally only patients with good oral hygiene are considered for orthodontic treatment but occasionally patients who would be better treated with fixed appliances are offered removable appliance treatment as a compromise because this makes it easier to maintain oral hygiene at an acceptable level. This is an unfortunate compromise as good oral hygiene is an essential prerequisite to any form of treatment with appliances.

Removable appliances should be taken out and brushed with soap and water and the mouth cleaned after every meal. Children should be encouraged to take a brush to school to clean teeth and appliance after the midday meal and at the very least the mouth and appliance should be rinsed with water at that time.

Diet should be that required for good general health and hard and sticky foods and sweets avoided

completely. It must be emphasized that appliances are worn at mealtimes, and this is particularly important when bite-planes are in use. The practice of removing appliances at mealtimes leads to carelessness in wearing the appliance at all, breakages and a falling off or failure of the treatment schedule.

Should problems occur with speech, bite-planes should be checked for height and width and if intrusion on space for the tongue is suspected, an appropriate adjustment should be made. If the appliance is comfortable, well fitting and does not constrict tongue movements, a good patient will have no problems with speech or eating.

Patients must be told quite clearly that if an appliance is causing pain or discomfort, they should attend the clinic at once and preferably not remove the appliance as it will then be possible to see what is causing the pain and take appropriate action. Patients should be advised not to persist with an appliance that is painful or uncomfortable in the belief that this is normal. To remove the appliance and wait is equally unsatisfactory as it may then not be possible to ascertain how the trouble arose and drifting of teeth may occur and the appliance cease to fit. If an appliance becomes painful and there is an insuperable difficulty in attending the clinic, then of course the appliance should be left out and a visit arranged at the earliest possible moment.

Patients should be instructed that in the event of breakage or loss of an appliance, they should return immediately bringing the broken appliance which it may be possible to repair. It is often useful to take an impression over a broken appliance to ensure that the fragments are in correct relation to one another and sometimes it is more satisfactory to reconstruct the appliance completely using some or all of the original clasps and springs. A lost appliance must, naturally, be replaced.

When the patient is familiar with the above rules and procedures for the management of his treatment, the parents, especially of young patients, should be fully informed of these details as well. Finally, if extractions are part of the treatment, parents should be asked to make an appointment with the family dentist or community clinic and a letter sent detailing the extractions to be done. The patient should be instructed to replace the appliance immediately after the extractions and an appointment made for appliance adjustment or to return sooner should any problem arise.

Subsequent visits

Patients wearing active removable appliances should be seen at monthly intervals. This is the period over which such appliances will continue to act and it is also wise to maintain contact and continuity with the patient. At subsequent visits the clinician should ascertain:

1. Is there cooperation – is the patient wearing and caring for the appliance as directed?
2. The degree of tooth movement – is the desired tooth movement taking place?

1. Proof that the appliance is being worn must be found and it is reasonable to ask whether the patient is wearing the appliance full-time. A casual enquiry as to how much the appliance is left out may actually reveal that it is removed at mealtimes or in language lessons or on some other occasions.

Examination of the appliance and the mouth will provide clues as to how things are going:

(a) the patient should be asked to remove and insert the appliance. Dexterity is to be expected if instructions are being carried out correctly;

(b) examination of the appliance out of the mouth should reveal a worn appearance of the baseplate such as faceting of bite-planes, loss of polish and possibly loss of small fragments at the edges;

(c) intra-oral examination may reveal a line demarcating the posterior border of the appliance on the palate and some imprint of the baseplate on the soft tissues;

(d) normal speech is to be expected after a period of continuous appliance wear and the persistence of lisping speech may suggest that the appliance is not being worn continuously. Bite-planes should be checked and adjusted if necessary so as to give the patient the best possible chance to adapt and speak normally.

The level of oral hygiene should be checked and advice and, if necessary, admonition given regarding the way the mouth and appliance are being cleaned. The patient should be asked if there are any problems or difficulties and appropriate help and advice given.

2. Tooth movement in the mouth can be assessed visually by comparison with the record casts of the original condition. Tooth movement can also be measured with calipers or dividers (*Figure 9.1*). In the case of distal movement of a maxillary canine measurement is made from the buccal groove of the upper first molar to the tip of the canine. Where the corresponding lower tooth is not being moved, changes in the occlusal relationship of the maxillary canine may be described in terms of premolar units.

Anchorage should be monitored at each visit so that undesirable movement of anchor teeth may be swiftly identified and additional anchorage provided, a reduction made in the number of teeth being moved or the amount of pressure adjusted.

Signs that anchorage is slipping may be identified by changes in occlusal relationships or changes in overjet (*Figure 9.2*). In the case of distal movement of upper buccal teeth, anchorage breakdown may show up in forward movement of upper molar teeth

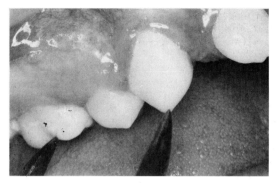

Figure 9.1 Measurement of distal movement of the upper canine using the buccal groove of the first permanent molar as a measuring point

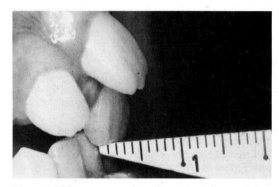

Figure 9.2 Measurement of overjet to check for possible slippage of anchorage

or by increase in overjet. It should be remembered that when an anterior bite-plane is used, bite opening may account for 1 mm increase in overjet due to backward rotation of the mandible. Increase in overjet of this order in these circumstances should not be viewed with alarm.

It should be borne in mind that the anchorage which may be derived from teeth becomes less with successive appliances as teeth which have recently been moved may have a tendency to relapse. This should be allowed for by over-correction of tooth position, adequate retention of teeth which have been recently moved and critical appraisal of anchorage requirements.

Extra-oral and functional appliances

It is a paradox that the management of part-time wearing of appliances should prove more fraught with problems than full-time wear. While full-time wear of such appliances would be desirable, these appliances fill the mouth, rendering eating, speech and participation in games impossible. Children of a shy and sensitive nature also dislike the unwelcome attention that headgear can attract.

Once again, children vary greatly and an enthusiastic patient can overcome all obstacles and wear these appliances virtually full-time while another patient may need considerable persuasion and convincing that the appliance must be worn at least in bed at night.

The term 'night time' should be dropped and, as a working rule, the patient should be advised that the more continuously the appliance is worn, the more quickly will the treatment be completed. He should be instructed that the appliance should be worn all the time when in the house at home but should not be taken outside the house.

The amount of time then available for appliance wearing will be considerable, from the time the patient comes home from school until leaving the following morning. This period will include time spent on homework, watching television, playing indoor games and recreations and in bed. Only mealtimes and oral hygiene need be deducted for functional appliances and the available time will be in excess of the 12–16 hours desired by many clinicians. At weekends and during holidays there will be even more time available. In short, the interested patient will find ways to keep his wearing time up and his treatment time down and such children relieve the clinician of a great deal of concern that his treatments will turn out well.

The reluctant patient is always a problem and time is well spent in encouraging such children to understand the need for their treatment and to desire improvement in their lot. Time sheets are a tangible way of keeping track of hours of wear and these should be carefully scrutinized at each visit. Clinicians should be aware that time sheets may be unreliable in many cases as shown by Clemmer and Hayes (1979), but knowledge of the patient and reference to the state of the appliance and the familiarity with which the patient assembles and inserts it together with the actual progress of treatment will help to expose the patient who 'cooks the books'.

It is important to emphasize the advantages of maximal wear to the reluctant patient and remind him of the opportunities provided by weekends and holidays to reduce the overall treatment time.

On the other hand, the over-zealous wearer of anchorage headgear may need to be watched and if necessary restrained to prevent the conversion of a Class II malocclusion into a Class III.

Retention

The stability of the dentition following the re-arrangements produced by orthodontic treatment depends mainly on the natural forces that remain acting on the crowns of the teeth and very little on what stability there may be in the periodontal tissues and bone surrounding the tooth roots after the teeth have settled down in their new positions. If there is an imbalance in the forces acting on the tooth crowns either from the soft-tissue environment or due to occlusal pressures, the teeth will change position after any retaining appliance has been removed. It is an important aspect of treatment planning to leave the teeth, after treatment, in positions that are inherently stable as far as can be foreseen.

An important point about retention is that retaining appliances should not continue to exert pressures on the teeth in the same way as appliances used for treatment. Retaining appliances should be rigid and simply hold the teeth in their new positions for a time to allow the periodontal tissues and bone to re-form about the tooth roots. An appliance used for treatment should not, therefore, be used for retention; a retention appliance such as a Hawley retainer should be used (*Figure 9.3*; Hawley, 1926) or active springs should be replaced by acrylic material or a rigid wire which simply maintains a tooth or a number of teeth in position without exerting pressure.

Because rearrangement of the teeth with removable appliances tends to be sequential rather than simultaneous, normally only the last tooth group moved should need to be retained. Where, for instance, the incisors have been aligned following retraction of premolars and canines, these latter teeth will have been held in position for periods upwards of six months and should be relatively stable.

Some treatment results have a high degree of stability, as for instance when an upper incisor tooth is moved labially across the bite and the degree of overbite is sufficient to ensure that the incisor will

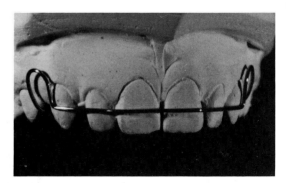

Figure 9.3 The Hawley retainer. The labial bow of 0.7 mm wire makes contact with the upper anterior teeth from canine to canine and the baseplate fits their lingual surfaces. Clasps on the first molars retain the appliance in position

not relapse. In such a case retention is hardly necessary.

Where all the teeth have been moved as in the treatment of postnormal occlusion using a functional appliance, it is a nice question as to what retention appliance should be used and for how long. An Andresen appliance with a working bite is an active appliance and for retention purposes an Andresen appliance with a bite taken in centric occlusion with the dental arches brought into contact will maintain the occlusion in the final treated relationship without exerting pressures and will act as a retainer which should be worn every night for three months and gradually reducing the number of nights per week for the following three months until the retainer is discarded.

The Kesling retainer (Kesling, 1945) made in a firm but slightly flexible inert material, i.e. a silastic silicon rubber or mouth-guard material, covers upper and lower dental arches and is constructed on casts placed in the final corrected occlusal relationship. Small displacements or rotations of individual teeth may be corrected by cutting off and repositioning the affected teeth on the casts before making the retainer. This appliance can be worn at night time or at times convenient to the patient in the same way as a functional appliance. Any final adjustments of tooth position are quite small and the material is stiff enough to act as a firm retainer and is managed and finally discarded in the same way as a conventional retaining appliance.

Long periods of retention are seldom justified and young patients especially should not be encumbered with retaining appliances for an indefinite future unless there are exceptional circumstances such as partial anodontia or a cleft palate problem. In older patients and, for instance, where periodontal treatment in conjunction with small tooth movements in the anterior region has been undertaken, stability may only be achieved by the use of a permanent retainer or by bonding a number of teeth together. In circumstances such as this the patient will fully understand the special hygiene measures needed to maintain such arrangements in a healthy condition.

At the completion of treatment, a final set of study casts should be made and during the retention period patients may be seen at longer intervals than during treatment. Continued attention should be paid to oral hygiene and the wearing of retaining appliances as instructed. Retaining appliances should be cared for and kept in as good condition as appliances used for treatment and repaired and adjusted when necessary.

Appendix A

Methods of wire forming

Wire may be formed in two ways. Firstly, special pliers may be used having grooves, nicks, serrations, additional parts attached and specially shaped beaks which by grasping the wire firmly create some special kind of bend. Such pliers relieve the user of the need for any particular skill in the manipulation of wire but this approach necessitates a number of pliers to meet the varying needs of appliance construction and adjustment.

Secondly, one very simple but strong and accurate plier may be used which makes it possible easily to hold the wire in an immovable grip with one hand. The required bend is then imposed on the wire with the thumb of the other hand. This second method has many advantages. The vast majority of wire-forming operations can be performed with one plier which becomes a Universal Plier; the strength and accuracy of such a plier makes it possible to form any wire used in orthodontic appliances including the heavier gauges used for extra-oral attachments.

For the formation of small coils in fine archwires and cantilever springs, pliers with òne square and one round beak will meet all needs from constructing self-supporting springs down to the finest finger springs.

Instruments for removable appliance construction and adjustment

Adams Universal Pliers and the principles of their use were conceived in 1946 and their specification published in 1950 as was a description of the fundamental principles of wire-forming using these pliers (Adams, 1950). In due course, a full specification was published (Adams, 1955). It is important that any pliers described as universal can be used to form any wire used in orthodontic appliances otherwise the description 'universal' cannot be correct.

Adams Universal Pliers

The essential features of these pliers are:

1. Adams Universal Pliers are made of a steel that is harder than the wires that they will be used to form.
2. The distance between the hinge pin and the tips of the beaks is short.
3. The handles are wide and comfortable to hold. The handles curve smoothly and prolonged use, as in the laboratory, does not fatigue or hurt the palm of the hand. The high ratio between the length of the handles and length of the beaks makes it easy to hold wire immovably in the pliers when forming a bend.
4. The shape of the beaks must be as shown in *Figures A1.1, A1.2 and A1.3*
5. The sides of the beaks must be flat.
6. The edges of the grasping surfaces of the beaks must be sharp and not bevelled or rounded.
7. The grasping surfaces of the beaks must be textured. These surfaces must not be polished but also must not be serrated or grooved. The finish left by grinding or filing is satisfactory, but today coating with tungsten dust is the finish of choice.
8. When the beaks are closed, the tips should be in contact but there should be a gap at the hinge tapering evenly to contact at the tips. The gap at the hinge should be 0.6 mm and a wire of this thickness must slide freely between the beaks at this point (*Figure A1.4*). This ensures that a 1.0 mm wire can be held firmly, the surfaces of the beaks then being parallel. When a wire is gripped at the tips of the beaks there is no tendency for the wire to slip out of the pliers. This is important in the construction of the Adams Clasp (*Figure A1.5*)

Many pliers resembling Universal Pliers have been manufactured and distributed but they do not

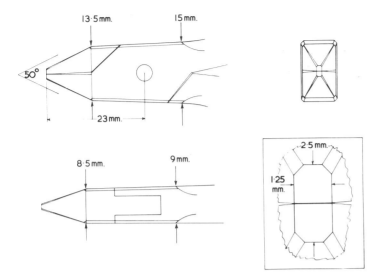

Figure A1.1 Adams Universal Pliers. The blades of these pliers must be accurately ground to the dimensions indicated. The tips of the beaks should not be less in size than shown

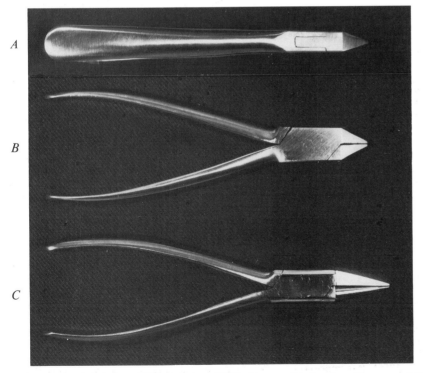

Figure A1.2 Adams Universal Pliers measure 5.25 inches overall in length and have gracefully curved handles designed for a maximum pressure with minimum expenditure of energy; *A*, the handles are comfortably broad to distribute the pressure over a wide area of the palm and fingers; *B*, the handles have a spread of 48 mm and the inner surfaces of the beaks taper to a gap of 0.6 mm at the hinge; *C*, spring-forming pliers have the same handles and hinge as Universal Pliers

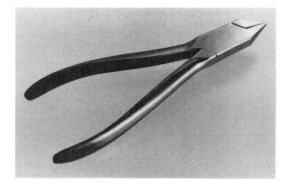

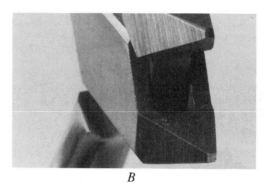

Figure A1.3 The general appearance of Adams Universal Pliers should bespeak the elegance, strength and accuracy of this instrument when correctly manufactured

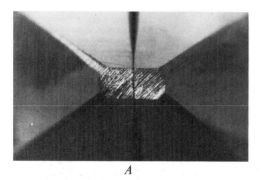

A

B

Figure A1.4 *A*, The tips of the pliers are ground very accurately to 1.0 mm square. The outer corners are slightly chamfered; *B*, the inner surfaces of the beaks are not polished, the edges of the beaks are quite sharp and must not be bevelled or rounded

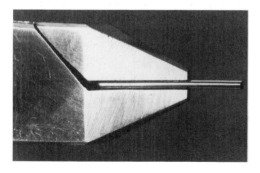

Figure A1.5 When a millimetre wire is grasped, the inside surfaces of the beaks are parallel

agree with the specification and are difficult or impossible to use. Faults commonly found in such pliers are:

1. The metal of the pliers is not hard enough. It is impossible to hold wire tightly with such pliers.
2. The construction is slender and wires of the thicker gauges cannot be grasped and formed.
3. Some manufacturers put a high polish on the pliers. If the grasping surfaces of the beaks are also polished, wires cannot be held with such surfaces.
4. The edges of the grasping surfaces are rounded or bevelled. These edges must be square and sharp so that wire can be held firmly and formed precisely.

5. The tips of the beaks are too large or too small.
6. The handles are not of the proper shape and size and cause fatigue and hurt to the hand in daily use. Handles are too long or too short and the pliers are then difficult to use.

Some of these faults can be remedied and some cannot. If the grasping surfaces of the beaks of the pliers are polished, the polish can be removed by grinding with a mounted stone in the handpiece. If the edges of the beaks are bevelled or rounded, the fault can be reduced by grinding the sides of the beaks on a grindstone (*Figures A1.6, A1.7* and *A1.8*).

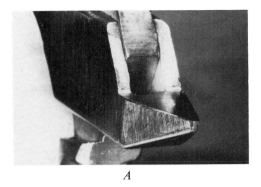
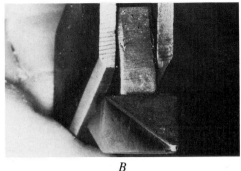

A

B

Figure A1.6 Faults in production; *A*, there is a polish on the grasping surfaces of the beaks and the edges are bevelled; *B*, the grasping surfaces of these pliers are correctly matt finished but there is a very large bevel on the grasping edges. Both these pliers are new and unused. The first pliers are virtually useless and the second pliers require correction before use

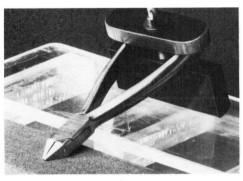
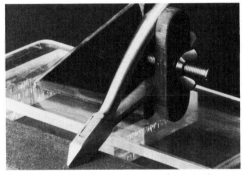

A

B

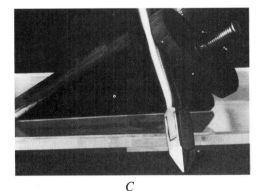

C

Figure A1.7 The correction and maintenance of Adams Universal Pliers; *A* and *B*, a general view of the jig and grindstone. The pliers are clamped, using the wing nuts, at correct angles for grinding; *C*, grinding the bevel on the outer edges of the beaks

Forming wire with Adams Universal Pliers

Wire is bent with Universal Pliers by holding it in the pliers in one hand and applying pressure with the thumb of the other hand, wrapping the fingers round the free end of the wire to aid complete control of the bend (*Figure A1.9A–C*).

Wire is never bent around the ends of Adams Universal Pliers. Wire is bent upon itself, using the properties of the wire to obtain the required form. Smooth curves are made in light wires such as are

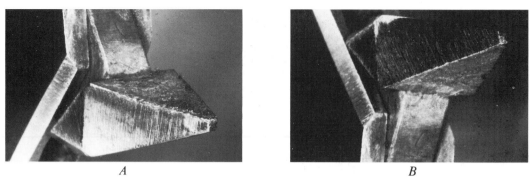

Figure A1.8 The correction of pliers that are bevelled or worn at the grasping edges; *A*, Adams Universal Pliers after some years of use. Note the turning over of the working edges; *B*, the same pliers after grinding the sides of the beaks. Note the straight sharp edge of the beak

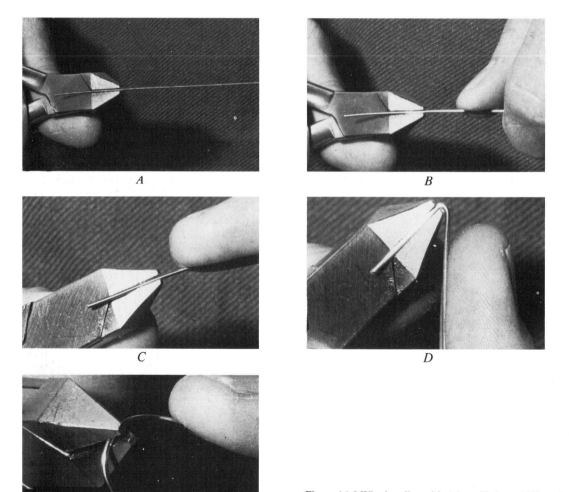

Figure A1.9 Wire bending with Adams Universal Pliers; *A*, the wire is held with an adequately long length projecting; *B–D*, wire may be bent easily by grasping the projecting length and applying pressure with the thumb; *E*, a large smooth bend is made up of a number of smaller bends

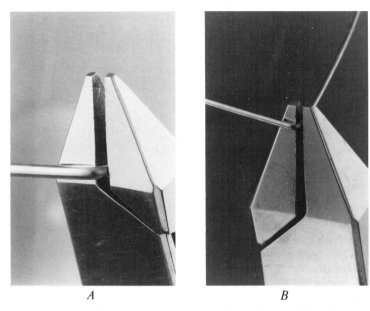

Figure A1.10 *A*, Making right angle bends with Adams Universal Pliers. Heavy wires are grasped close to the hinge and bent through 90°; *B*, lighter wires can similarly be bent nearer to the tips of the pliers

used in multiband orthodontic appliances by holding the end of the archwire in the pliers and 'wiping' a bend into the wire using the thumb of the other hand. The same can be done with heavier wires used for labial and lingual arches in removable appliances.

Smooth bends are made in any gauge of orthodontic wire by making a series of small bends, adding them into a gentle bend up to a full circle. Such bends are used for circular extra-oral hooks and for U loops in labial arches (*Figure A1.9E*).

Right angle bends are made by laying the wire

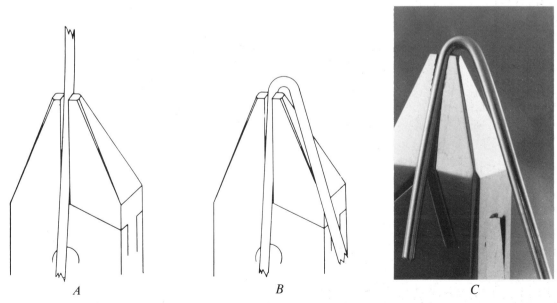

Figure A1.11 Making an acute bend in a heavy wire; *A*, the wire is held obliquely in the pliers; *B*, the wire is bent over the tip of the pliers and not round the tip. Holding the wire as shown ensures that an immovable grip of the wire is obtained; *C*, photograph of a completed bend made in this way

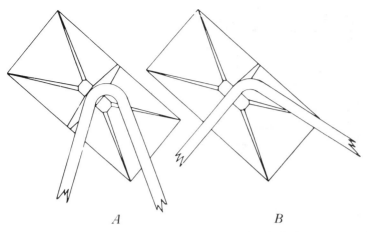

A   *B*

Figure A1.12 The correction of sharp bends in heavy wire; *A*, the incorrect part of the bend is grasped in the tips of Adams Universal Pliers and squeezed firmly; *B*, this will straighten this portion of the wire. The sharp edges of the beaks prevent the wire from slipping, but do not injure the wire. The wire is then bent where required

across the beaks of the pliers, holding and bending through a right angle. Light wires are bent near the tips of the beaks, heavier wires nearer to the hinge where a stronger grip can be obtained *Figure A1.10A and B*).

Acute bends are made in two ways depending on the thickness of the wire. Heavy wires are first bent to a right angle as described. The wire is then laid obliquely along the length of the beaks so that the full length of the beaks is used to hold the wire which is then bent over the tips of one beak into an angle of the required acuteness (*Figure A1.11A–C*). If it is required that this angle should be closed so that the limbs lie parallel, the bend is compressed between the beaks of the pliers.

If the wire is bent at a slightly incorrect position, a correction may be made if the wire is straightened as shown in *Figure A1.12*. The incorrect portion of the bend is gripped in the tips of the pliers and squeezed. This has the effect of straightening the small section of wire without interfering with the remainder of the bend. The wire is then bent at the correct point.

An efficient and trouble-free extra-oral hook can be made in any heavy wire by making a right angle and an acute angle bend as shown in *Figure A1.13*. The operation takes about five or six seconds to complete and no specialized pliers are required.

Acute bends are made in fine wires as for Adams clasps or for U loops in light archwires by first making a right angle bend. The wire is then held in the tips of the beaks of the pliers and the wire is bent through a second right angle as shown in *Figure A1.14*. Note that the wire is not bent round the tip of the beaks but between the beaks.

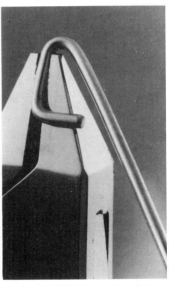

Figure A1.13 The formation of a hook on extra-oral 'whiskers'. A right angle and an acute angle bend produce a hook to which elastics can easily be attached and which will not catch in bed clothing

Orthodontic technique exercises

Skill in wire-forming can quickly be gained by the use of simple geometrical exercises using wire 1.0 mm thick. The first exercise consists of bending wire so as to fit round two rows of pins in a zigzag manner. This requires accurate placing of sharp

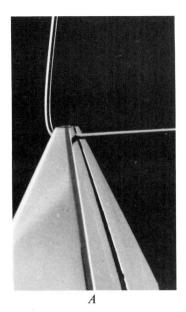
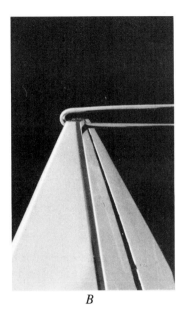

A   B

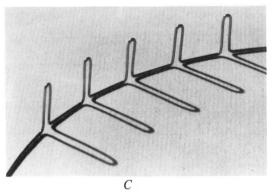

C

Figure A1.14 Making acute bends in fine wires. A right angle bend is first made and the wire held as shown in *A*; the wire is then bent through a further right angle so making a U. Note that the wire is not bent round the beaks of the pliers but outside and between the beaks as at *B*; using this method it is possible to form a multi-loop light archwire, *C*.

turns in the wire and the method of adjusting the position of a sharp turn in a heavy wire may be needed.

At first no attempt should be made to fit the wire exactly round the pins. It is more important to ensure that the wire lies flat and does not bind on the pins. As confidence is gained further samples should be made to fit the wire more accurately while ensuring that it lies flat and is not tight on the pins (*Figure A1.15A* and *B*). The second exercise, consisting of six square pegs, makes use of the principle of working wire into corners or angles between objects as shown in the illustration (*Figure A1.15C*). *Figure A1.15D–G* shows four further exercises designed to inculcate other aspects of wireforming skills.

Adams Spring-Forming Pliers

Adams Spring-Forming Pliers are constructed to the same physical and ergonomic standards as Adams Universal Pliers. On taking these pliers in the hand, the sensation is identical but the elegant beaks, designed for loop and coil forming, indicate the purpose of the instrument (*Figure A1.17*).

Adams Spring-Forming Pliers make possible the forming of loops and coils in the thinnest and the thickest wires used for orthodontic appliance construction.

It is important to respect the construction of the pliers and not to attempt to bend thick wires at a point too close to the ends of the beaks. If this principle is borne in mind, thick wires may be formed close to the hinge and the finer wires formed towards the ends of the beaks.

Adams Spring-Forming Pliers are used in the same manner as Adams Universal Pliers. The smoothly-formed handles make it easy to grasp a wire with one hand and wrap the wire round the conical beak of the pliers with the thumb of the other hand into a half-round loop or a circular coil of the desired size (*Figures A1.17* and *A1.18*).

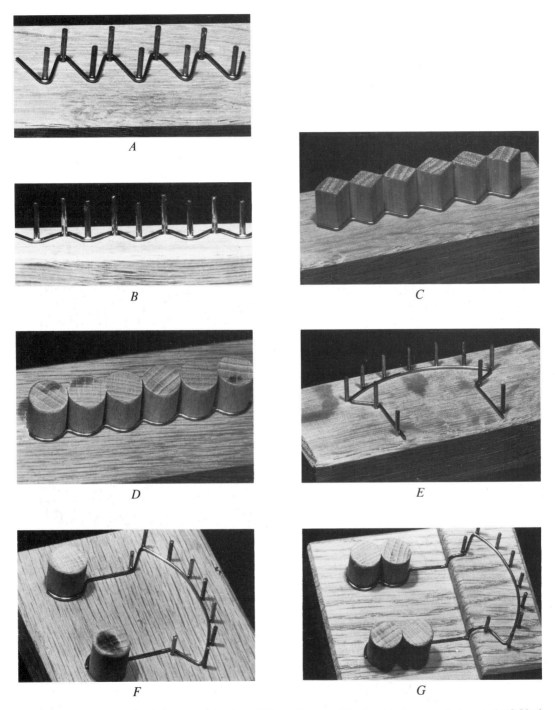

Figure A1.15 *A*, Exercise No. 1: the pins are hard steel 1.0 mm thick set 0.5 inch apart, the rows of pins are also 0.5 inch apart; *B*, this illustration shows that the wire must be flat at all points on the wood block; *C*, exercise No. 2: the posts are square and 0.5 inch in diagonal. The corners against which the wire is fitted are very slightly rounded, it being impossible to make a perfectly sharp angle in 1.0 mm wire; *D*, exercise No. 3: the posts are 0.5 inch in diameter and 0.5 inch high; *E*, exercise No. 4: simple lingual arch prototype; *F*, exercise No. 5: lingual arch prototype. The posts are 0.5 inch in diameter; *G*, exercise No. 6: difficult lingual arch prototype. The step in the block makes the arch three-dimensional. The step is 0.25 inch deep, the posts are 0.5 inch in diameter

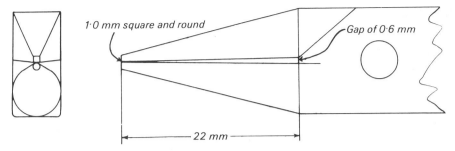

Figure A1.16 Spring-forming pliers should be accurately ground to the dimensions shown. The tips should be at most 1.0 mm square and round in size, but may be less if desired and the quality of the metal will permit

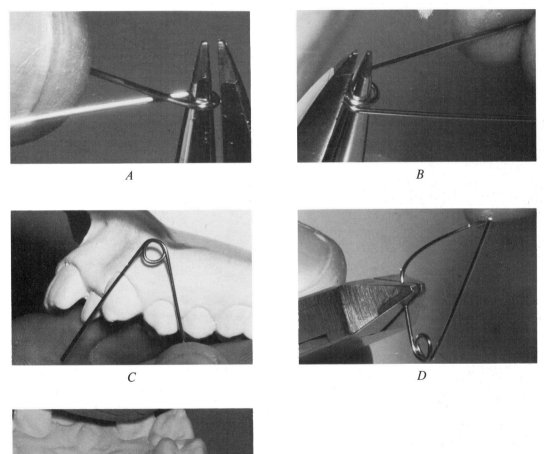

Figure A1.17 Using Adams Spring-Forming Pliers for bending medium gauge wire; forming a canine retractor of 0.7 mm wire: *A* and *B*, making the coil. Note that the thumb is used for bending the wire; *C*, trying the spring in place; *D*, bending the tag over into the palate – Adams Universal Pliers are better for this; *E*, the tag is finished as before. Note that the free end of the spring is left as in *C* or a little shorter and is finished and fitted in the clinic. If desired, however, this fitting can be done in the laboratory

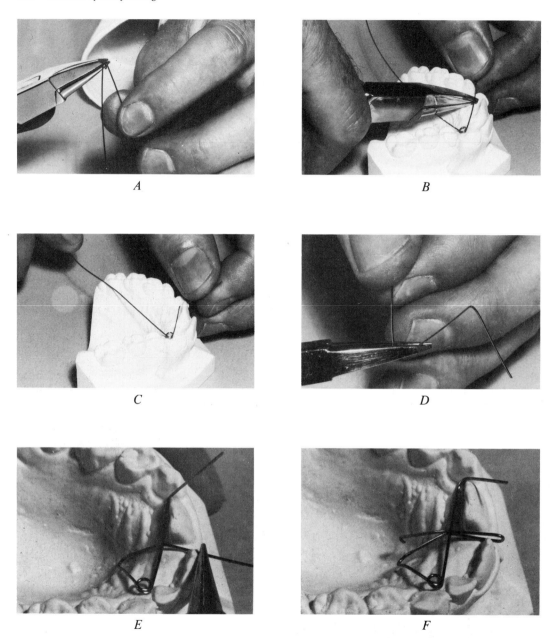

Figure A1.18 Manipulating fine wire with spring-forming pliers. Making a finger spring of 0.5 mm wire to procline an upper incisor tooth. *A*, A single coil is placed in the wire; *B*, the spring is tried in place and the free end marked by grasping in the pliers; *C*, the free end is turned round the tooth to be moved; *D*, the tag end is turned down into the palate at the coil and brought back again across the spring to form the guide; *E*, the guide is marked for length by grasping with the pliers and turned back into the palate so completing the tag; *F*, the completed spring. Note that the guide is carried well forward and passes between the central incisors, there being a space between these teeth

Appendix B

The Adams Clasp, construction and adjustment

Construction of the clasp

Preparation of the plaster cast

In orthodontic patients the gum margins of the permanent teeth have not usually fully receded to the anatomical necks. It is therefore necessary, on the dental cast, to trim the interdental papillae so that the mesial and distal undercuts are made accessible on the teeth to be clasped. This is best done with a very sharp chisel about 3 mm wide. Wax carvers and knives are not suitable for this operation – only a chisel will do.

The preparation of the cast is important and it is necessary to reproduce the subgingival shape of the tooth accurately. There must be no exaggeration of the undercuts and holes must not be made in the plaster cast mesially and distally to the tooth being clasped (*Figure B1.1*).

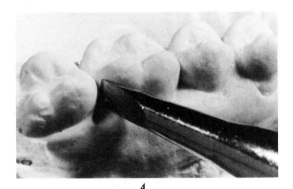

A

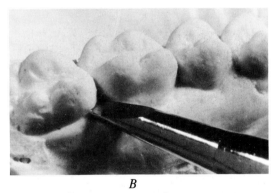

B

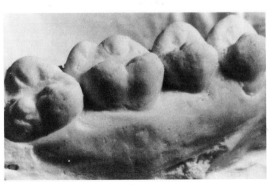

C

Figure B1.1 Trimming the plaster tooth for fitting the Adams Clasp; *A*, a broad enamel chisel is laid against the tooth and the plaster cut vertically; *B*, the enamel chisel is laid horizontally and plaster removed to show the undercut of the tooth; *C*, the appearance of the tooth after the trimming is complete

Formation of the Adams Clasp

For molar and premolar teeth and for deciduous teeth, 0.7 mm hard stainless steel wire (120–130 tons per sq in tensile strength) is used. For canine teeth, 0.6 mm wire is used. A piece of wire 7–8 cm long is sufficient.

There are three stages in the formation of an Adams Clasp (*Figure B1.2*) and each arrowhead is made by three distinct bends, as follows:

1. The first bend is of a little more than a right angle. Two such bends are made, connected by a bridge sufficiently long to span the tooth that is being clasped (*Figure B1.3A and B and Figure B1.2, no. 1*).

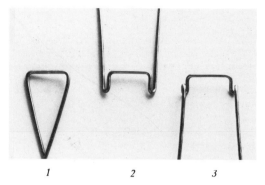

1   *2*   *3*

Figure B1.2 Stages in bending the clasp

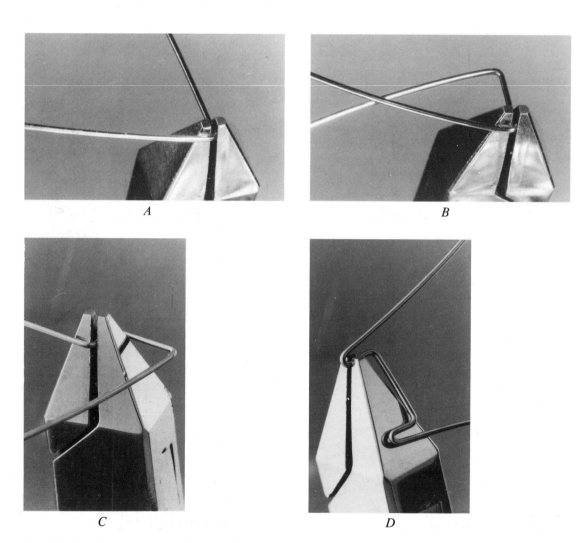

A

B

C

D

Figure B1.3 Bending the arrowhead clasp; *A* and *B*, two bends made of a little more than 90°; *C*, the formation of the arrowhead. The wire is first bent at right angles; *D*, the clasp is tilted downwards against the pliers and the arrowhead formed by bending outside the tip of the beak.

2. The second bend (*Figure B1.2, no. 2*) is made in two stages of 90° each as shown in *Figure B1.3C and D*. This second bend forms a U turn in the wire of 180°, made outside the tips of the pliers so that a tight, acute bend is formed, the sides of the resulting arrowhead being parallel. The arrowheads may be squeezed slightly in the pliers to make them neater if necessary (*Figure B1.3E*).

Three checks and adjustments are now made to the arrowheads. First the slope of the arrowheads is adjusted to follow the gum margins (*Figure B1.3F and G*); second, the arrowheads are made parallel if they are not already so (*Figure B1.2, no. 2*); third, the clasp is tried on the tooth to check that the width is correct (*Figure 1.3H*).

It should be noted that there is no absolutely fixed width of clasp for any given tooth or any tooth measurement that helps in deciding how long the bridge of the clasp should be. The bridge must not be so long that the arrowheads touch the adjoining teeth. If the bridge is too short and the arrowheads are too close together they will impinge on the buccal surface of the tooth rather than on the mesial and distal undercuts. There is a degree of permissible variability in the width of the clasp. This variability is greater for molar teeth than it is for premolar teeth which have narrow necks.

It should also be noted that the bridge of the clasp should be straight; the bridge must not be bent to adjust the fit of the clasp.

3. The third bend brings the tags of the clasp over the embrasure between the teeth and onto the lingual side of the dental arch to be embedded in the baseplate material. To make the third bend, the arrowhead is grasped from the inside of the clasp with half of the length of the arrowhead between the beaks of the pliers. The tag is then bent firmly upwards, using the thumb, and the bend continued until the tag is at a little less than 90° to the arrowhead (*Figure B1.4A and B*).

Note that in making this bend, the wire is not bent over the beak of the pliers but is bent outside the tip as can be seen in *Figure B1.4*.

When this bend has been made, the clasp is tried on the tooth to check the angulation of the arrowheads to the tooth and the direction the tag is taking to the groove between the marginal ridges of the teeth (*Figure B1.4C*). Any necessary adjustments are made and the second tag is bent in a similar way.

The clasp is completed by bending the tags over the contact point between two teeth, into the lingual embrasures and then to bend the wire slightly away

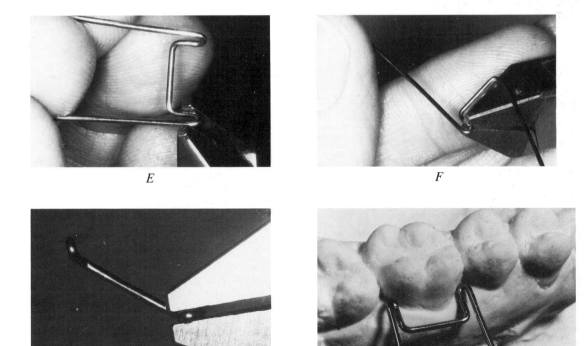

E

F

G

H

Figure B1.3 continued The second arrowhead is formed in the same way; *E*, the arrowheads are squeezed slightly; *F* and *G*, the arrowheads are aligned to follow the contours of the gum; *H*, the clasp is tried on the tooth

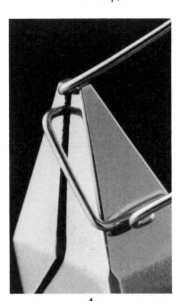

A

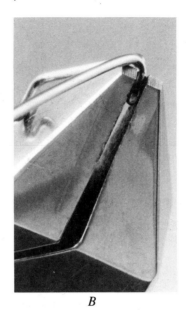

B

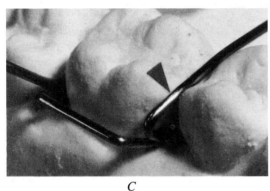

C

Figure B1.4 Details of formation of the tags; *A* and *B*, the arrowhead is grasped from inside the clasp and the tag is bent through 90°. Holding the arrowhead at the tip of the pliers, the tag is bent through a further 45° and then tried on the tooth, as at *C*, before completing the tag. The arrow indicates the point at which a slight bend is made to tension the clasp

from the palatal mucosa and turn the ends of the tags towards the palate and cut off leaving a small turn-down of 1–1.5 mm. This will ensure that the clasp is stabilized while the baseplate is being constructed and the tags are embedded securely in the baseplate material.

Figure B1.5A–D illustrates the features of the Adams Clasp and these pictures should be studied carefully to see exactly how the tags of the clasp are fitted, where they cross the occlusal plane and how the arrowheads and the bridge are placed in relation to the tooth.

Essential features of the Adams Clasp

1. The bridge is straight, not curved or bent. The bridge stands clear of the tooth and of the gum as shown in *Figure B1.5A–C*. The bridge is not fitted against the buccal surface of the tooth.

2. The arrowheads are parallel as shown in *Figure B1.5A* and do not converge or diverge.

3. The arrowheads slope to correspond with the curve of the gum margin into the interdental papilla. The arrowheads are not twisted into a vertical plane or laid in a horizontal plane (*Figure B1.5B*).

4. The tags fit closely across the contact point and are brought down into the interdental embrasure lingually so as to avoid the bite of the opposing teeth as shown in *Figure B1.5C* and *D*. The ends of the tags are supported by turning down at the ends leaving a clear space between the tag and the plaster cast. This ensures secure embedding of the tags in the baseplate.

5. Loops and extravagant lateral bends in the tags are unnecessary, wasteful of time and much less efficient than the finish shown in *Figure B1.5D*.

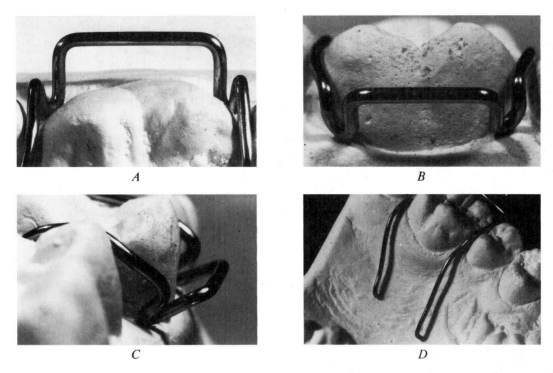

Figure B1.5 The essential features of the Adams Clasp; *A*, the bridge is straight. The sides of each arrowhead are parallel and the arrowheads are parallel to one another. The bridge stands away from the tooth, the arrowheads do not touch the adjoining teeth; *B*, the arrowheads slope to match the contour of the gum; *C*, the bridge stands clear from the tooth and half way between the tooth and the gum surface. The tags arch over the contact points; *D*, the tags are quite simply formed by turning down at right angles to the palate. A uniform space is left under the tags to encase them in the baseplate material

Adjustment of the Adams Clasp

It is important to distinguish between fitting clasps and adjusting clasps because there sometimes seems to be confusion between the two operations.

Clasps are made to fit at the time of construction. If clasps do not fit when an appliance is placed in the mouth, is is most unlikely that they can be made to fit by attempting to modify the shape of the clasps while the tags are embedded in the baseplate.

Adjusting a clasp is a totally different operation from fitting a clasp. Adjustment takes but a moment and consists of making one slight bend at each tag. This adjusts the amount of grip that the clasp exerts.

If the tags are not fitted closely in contact with the teeth and into the lingual embrasure, the appliance will be most uncomfortable to wear and will move or bounce when the patient closes the teeth together.

Failure of clasps to fit when a new appliance is placed in position must be attributed to an incorrect working cast or to poor construction of the clasp. All appliances should be delivered to the clinic on the casts on which they were constructed. If the clasps fit the cast but do not fit the patient then the impression must be faulty or damaged in pouring the cast.

Much misunderstanding and trouble arises from the belief that Adams Clasps need to be fitted in the clinic. If clasps do not fit when a new appliance is placed, then a further appliance should be insisted on.

Adams Clasps are constructed so that the arrowheads fit against the mesial and distal under-cuts on the tooth. The clasp does not necessarily exert a grip on the natural tooth when the appliance has been processed. If the clasp does grip the tooth, this means that too much plaster was trimmed away when preparing the cast for clasp construction. At the time of placing the appliance the clasps should just make contact with the teeth or exert a very slight grip.

The clasps are then adjusted to obtain the desired degree of grip by bending the arrowheads very slightly towards the tooth. The point in the tags where this adjusting bend is made is shown clearly in *Figures B1.4* and *B1.6*. It should be noted carefully that the adjusting bend is made buccally to where the tag makes contact with the teeth in crossing the

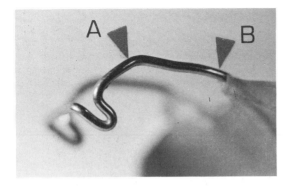

Figure B1.6 The tag of an Adams Clasp indicating where a slight bend should be made at A, just buccally to the embrasure between the teeth, to tension the clasp. Adjustment of the clasp for tension is not made at any other point on the tag and must not be made at point B

teeth in crossing the contact point. The manner of making the adjustment is shown in *Figure B1.7.*

Bends should not be made in tags where they emerge from the baseplate (*Figure B1.6*), as this will prevent a well-fitting appliance with well-fitting clasps from seating properly in the mouth. If the clasp does not fit properly, bending the tags where they emerge from the baseplate will not make the clasp fit. It is only possible to adjust the grip of a clasp if the clasp fits correctly in the first place.

Conclusions

The Adams Clasp should be made and used exactly as described when it will meet every requirement. It is possible to form hooks as part of the clasp for intermaxillary traction and to construct the clasp for deciduous teeth and for upper permanent canine teeth (*Figure B1.8*). Tubes can also be soldered to the bridges of clasps for extra-oral attachments (*see Figures 7.7 and C1.11*). In every case the basic form

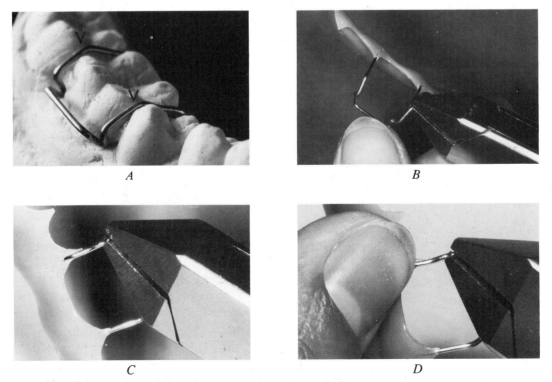

Figure B1.7 Adjusting the Adams Clasp; *A*, the bends are made just beyond the point where the tag bends down towards the arrowhead; *B*, the position at which the tag is held for adjusting the clasp; *C* and *D*, the same

of the clasp is maintained so that clasping efficiency is undiminished.

From time to time attempts are made to modify the Adams Clasp by placing the arrowheads horizontally or vertically instead of aligned with the curve of the gum margins or by allowing the bridge to make contact with the neck of the tooth. Clasps are sometimes made to span two teeth. Clasps which exhibit these characteristics are not Adams Clasps or even variations of Adams Clasps as they are sometimes called, and cannot work as well as the original design. The Adams Clasp is designed to clasp a single tooth and works most efficiently in this way.

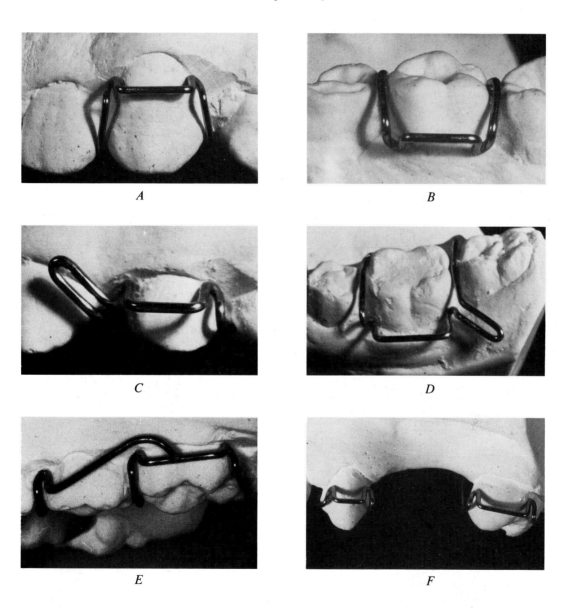

Figure B1.8 *A*, The Adams Clasp on the upper permanent canine. The wire is 0.6 mm for this purpose; *B*, the clasp on a lower second deciduous molar, the wire is 0.7 mm. Sometimes deciduous teeth are very short in the crown and the clasp has to be very flat; *C* and *D*, traction hooks on upper premolar and lower molar. In the lower molar it is possible simply to weld a hook of 0.7 mm soft stainless steel wire onto the bridge if required; *E*, the accessory arrowhead clasp. This is most conveniently welded to the bridge of the main clasp which is a far better arrangement than the practice of bridging two teeth by the same clasp. If either tooth moves even slightly, the clasp ceases to work properly; *F*, clasping teeth in which there is gum recession. The full depth of the undercut must never be used otherwise the clasp will be totally ineffective;

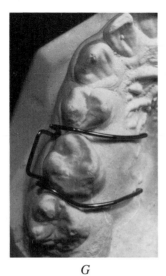

G

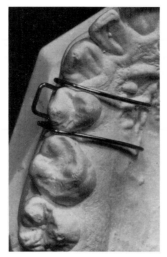

H

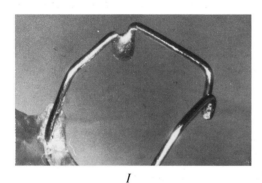

I

Figure B1.8 continued *G* and *H*, clasps on rotated teeth. The clasp should be made in the usual way and the bridge should be in line with the buccal segment and not with the buccal surface of the rotated tooth; *I*, a soldered repair of the arrowhead of a clasp

Appendix C

Welding and soldering for orthodontic appliance construction

Joints can be made in stainless steel by spot welding or by soldering. Welds are made by passing an electric current through the pieces to be joined which are simultaneously pressed together. The current heats the metal which becomes plastic and the pressure forges the softened metals into a single piece. Soldering entails heating the metals to be joined in a flame and applying a solder or brazing compound which encases the pieces to be joined. Oxidization of the solder and metal is prevented by the use of a flux.

Welding for appliance construction

The orthodontic welder

A welder consists of an electric transformer which reduces the voltage of the mains supply to a low value which is safe to handle, copper electrodes which convey the current to the workpieces, a pressure mechanism to keep the workpieces pressed into contact and a timing switch to control the duration of current flow. As a rule the working voltage is also variable by means of tappings on the primary circuit of the transformer and power input on the primary side may be adjusted by a variable resistance (*Figure C1.1*)

The heat generated in metal when a current is passed through it is expressed by the formula

$$H \propto I^2 RT$$

where H is heat in joules, I is current in amperes, R is resistance in ohms, T is duration of current in seconds. In lowering the voltage in the welding circuit, the transformer correspondingly makes available a high current which, it can be seen from the formula, contributes greatly to the generation of heat which is proportional to the square of the

current, the resistance of the material and the time for which the current flows.

When a weld is made, the point of highest resistance is at the place where the workpieces are pressed into contact and in the workpieces themselves, which have a high resistance. The copper electrodes have low resistance, little heat is generated in them and having a high specific heat value, temperature rise is very small (*Figure C1.2*).

The main heating takes place between the workpieces which soften and are welded together by the pressure of the electrodes.

Figure C1.3 illustrates a simple orthodontic welder with a manual timing switch.

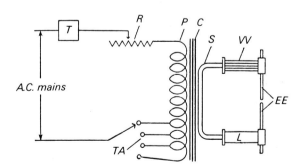

Figure C1.1 The electrical circuit of a spot welder; P, the primary winding of the transformer; C, core of the transformer; T, the timing switch; S, secondary winding of the transformer; TA, tappings on the primary winding; R, a variable resistance; VV, flexible springs which conduct current to the upper electrode and exert pressure on the workpieces; L, the lower electrode holder; EE, the electrodes

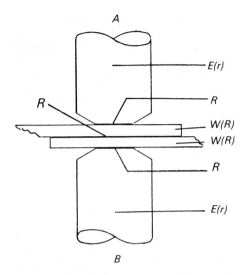

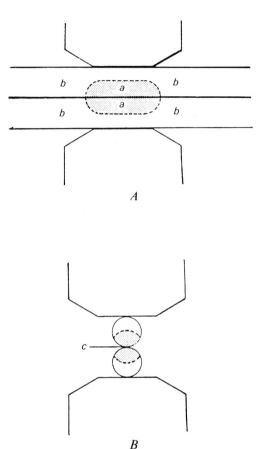

Figure C1.2 Variation in the resistance between the electrodes. The electrodes *EE* have small resistances, *rr*. The workpieces *WW* have large resistances, *RR*. The resistance between the workpieces is higher than at any other point in the circuit and it is here that the highest temperature is created. Although there is some heat developed between the electrodes and the workpieces, this heat is quickly dispersed in the electrodes which have a high specific heat

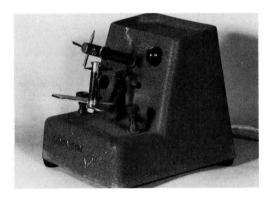

Figure C1.3 This is a fairly simple portable orthodontic welder. The switch is manual and the electrodes are of the turret type giving a choice of pairs for different purposes

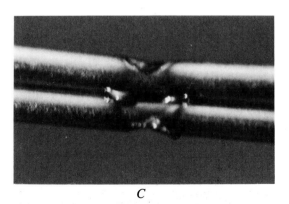

Welding orthodontic materials

Soft flat stainless steel, formerly used for orthodontic bands, can be welded very easily and while bonding and preformed bands have replaced band construction in the surgery, in removable appliance construction it is useful to be able to attach fine wires, as for apron springs, to heavy archwires by means of loops of narrow stainless steel tape.

Figure C1.4 The welding of wires; *A*, if the wires are laid parallel and flat electrodes are used, heating occurs in the area *a,a*. Softening should not penetrate more than four-fifths of the thickness of the wires. Support at *b,b,b,b* of unsoftened wire prevents fusion of the softened areas into a weld nugget; *B*, cross section of the resulting weld shows how very little fusion of metal can take place in such circumstances; *C*, increasing the welding current produces burning of the wire without improving the weld

The welding of soft stainless steel wires is not difficult but the welding of hard wires to one another requires some care as such wires are weakened by heat and a joint that is over-welded is not safe.

If wires are laid parallel to one another, the welding current is dispersed on either side of the point of weld and a poor join is made. If the current or welding time is increased, damage begins to take place to the outer surfaces of the wire where the electrodes make contact (*Figure C1.4*).

The correct answer to this problem is to weld wires at right angles to one another and to groove the electrodes so that the welding current is spread over a wider area of the outer surface of the wires than if the electrodes are flat. This method avoids damage to the wires and concentrates the welding effort at the point where the wires cross. A single, completely controlled weld can then be made (*Figure C1.5*). This method is particularly necessary when welding a thinner wire to a thicker one (*Figure C1.6*). For very fine wires the method of attaching fine wires by tape is better (*Figure C1.7*).

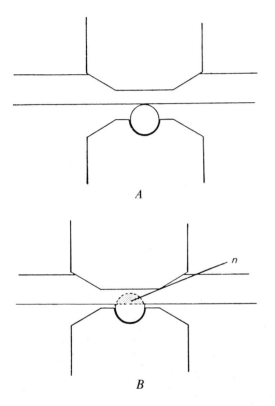

A

B

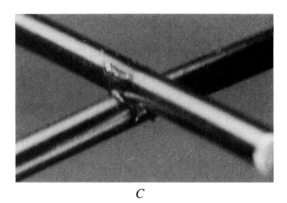

C

Figure C1.5 Welding wires at right angles using grooved electrodes; *A*, before welding; *B*, after welding. Note how the groove protects the outer surface of the wire and how all heating and fusion take place at the point of contact of the wires which sink into one another forming a weld nugget, *n*; *C*, the contours of the wires are protected and the weld is made between the contact surfaces of the wires

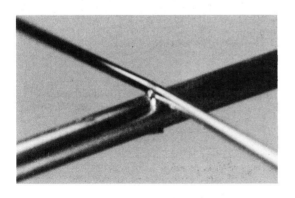

Figure C1.6 A fine wire welded to a thick wire. By using grooved electrodes and laying the wires at right angles the weld is confined to the contact area between the wires and the outer contours are not damaged

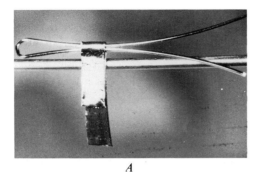

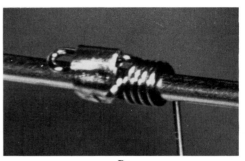

A   B

Figure C1.7 The welded tape loop for attaching fine spring wires; *A*, a loop of tape 2.5 mm × 0.15 mm is pulled up tightly on the fine spring wire. The tape loop is welded to the heavy archwire. The tape loop is cut off and welded to the arch again close up to but not through the spring wire. The wire loop is then pulled by the short end into the tape loop until jamming occurs and the short tail of wire turned tightly back; *B*, the short tail is cut off and smoothed, the tape welds and cut ends are smoothed and the spring is wound. Note how the pull of winding the spring is against the loop of tape and not against the weld. This attachment is suitable for any fine apron spring. Even when coils are not wanted, one or two turns of the spring wire are taken around the arch

Soldering for removable appliance construction

Soldering is a traditional method for joining metals used in orthodontics and suitable solder and flux are avaiable for stainless steel.

Equipment and materials

A miniature blowlamp run on propane or butane gas as used by jewellers is satisfactory for orthodontic soldering and if the flame is adjustable, a small quiet flame will be found to be more controllable than an over-hot flame (*Figure C1.8*).

Special solder wire and flux are necessary for stainless steel and these are available with other orthodontic materials. Solder does not unite with stainless steel so that, to ensure a satisfactory joint, the workpieces should be encased in solder and care taken not to overheat the soldering operation. If a joint is well made the surface of the solder will be smooth and polishing should not be necessary as this will thin or completely remove the solder coat and weaken the joint.

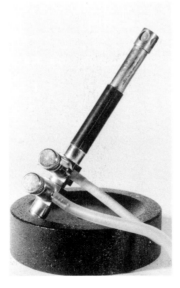

Figure C1.8 A jeweller's blowlamp for butane gas and low pressure air gives a fine, hot and controllable flame which is ideally suited for orthodontic soldering

Methods

Much orthodontic soldering is done freehand and as it is difficult to hold two wires and the solder wire in the flame simultaneously it is a good idea to coat one of the wires with sufficient solder for the whole joint first of all. It is then only necessary to melt the solder and place the second wire in the pool of melted solder when union will take place.

Stainless steel soldering requires very generous use of flux to prevent the formation of oxides which spoil the joint.

Wires of the same thickness present no problem in soldering but if one wire is much thinner than the other care must be taken not to overheat the finer wire.

A thinner wire may be wound round a thicker wire before soldering and this makes a very strong joint (*Figure C1.9*). A very thin wire may be wound round a thicker wire and solder flowed onto the joint from a third wire on which solder has been melted (*Figure C1.10*).

Tubes may be soldered to the bridges of Adams Clasps on molars or premolars for extra-oral

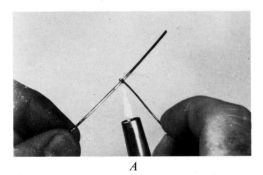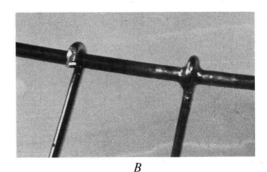

Figure C1.9 Soldering a thinner wire to a thicker one; *A*, the thinner wire is wound round the thicker wire first of all; *B*, the joint before and after soldering

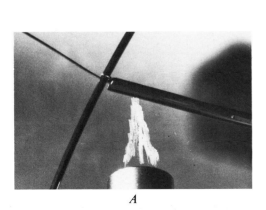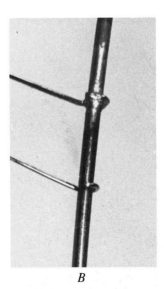

Figure C1.10 Soldering a very thin wire to a thick wire; *A*, a soldering iron of thick copper wire is used; *B*, a joint before and after soldering

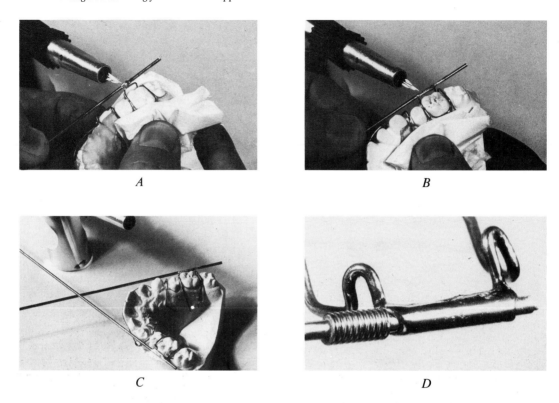

Figure C1.11 Soldering tubes; *A*, the tubing is coated with an adequate amount of solder; *B*, the flame is applied to the tube and the clasp is moved up against the molten solder which flows around it; *C*, both tubes have been soldered; the first tube is used as a guide for the second; *D*, the completed tube showing an archwire with a friction-fit stop

attachments. In making this joint, the arrowheads, tags and baseplate should be protected with damp paper. Solder is melted onto the tubing first and while this solder is held molten, the bridge of the clasp is laid in contact with the molten solder which rapidly encases the bridge creating a strong, smooth joint which does not need to be polished (*Figure C1.11*) (*see also Figure 7.7*).

The best joints for tubes are made freehand. Tacking the tube in place with a weld first of all or with a loop of tape is not a good idea as this forms oxides and creates interstices into which solder may not flow. The result is usually neither a good weld nor a good soldered joint. A well-made freehand soldered joint will not break down.

Appendix D

The orthodontic study cast

Study casts are essential records and a quick and routine method of producing casts from record impressions is a vital necessity.

Impressions for records should extend to the limit of the buccal sulcus in the upper and lower arches but should not extend beyond the hard palate and should include a good impression of the lingual sulcus in the molar region of the lower arch. All too often impressions are short in the upper and lower labial sulci and hardly ever extend into the lingual sulcus in the lower molar area. The resulting record casts show little more than the crowns of the teeth.

The bases of study casts should be of uniform height and symmetrical outline and should come into correct occlusion when placed with the heels down on a flat surface and gently brought into contact. Casts which are not finished in this way have to be brought into occlusion experimentally and freehand and there is too much scope for damage to the teeth rendering the casts unreliable as records.

Equipment

The equipment required includes a plaster cutting machine, rubber boxes for pouring casts, a T piece of firm rubber about 5 mm thick, a simple engineer's scribing block, a symmetroscope and three aligning jigs of 3 mm perspex (*Figures D1.1, D1.2* and *D1.3*).

A single, general purpose grinding machine will suffice unless the casts are needed for display when a second cutter with a fine-grit wheel is useful to give a smooth finish to the cut surfaces.

While the outline of the casts can be cut freehand, it is easier to produce uniform results by the use of a jig or guide to fix the angle for each side of the casts. Some cutters have an adjustable fence for this purpose.

Materials and methods

Record impressions should be cast in rubber moulds giving bases adequate for subsequent trimming with a plaster grinder. White plaster of good quality, if properly mixed and cast, is adequate for study casts which should in any case be handled with care and properly stored. Stone plaster may be used if desired but creates more expense and trouble.

The casts should be registered with a wax bite, taken in the clinic at the same time as the record impressions. The wax bite should consist of a small softened roll of wax placed transversely just behind the canine teeth and bitten into by the patient. Too large and bulky a bite registration separates the teeth. Most of the back teeth should be in contact without an intervening layer when the wax registration is made otherwise the occlusion of the teeth with the wax bite in place will be different from that when the registration is removed.

The stages of trimming the bases of record casts are shown in *Figures D1.4–D1.25*. For everyday use smoothing and filling the cut surfaces of the bases may be omitted.

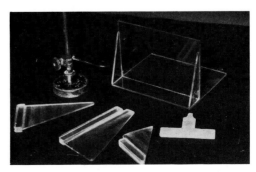

Figure D1.1 The surface gauge, symmetroscope, set squares and the rubber T piece

177

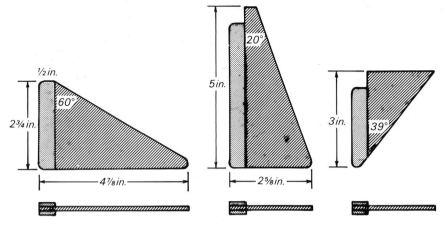

Figure D1.2 The set squares for trimming study models. These are made to the shapes and sizes shown in perspex cemented with chloroform

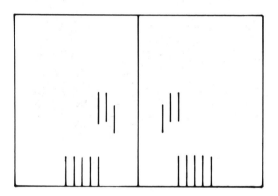

Figure D1.3 The screen of the symmetroscope measures 15 × 10 cm. The markings are 5 mm apart and are distributed symmetrically about the centre line

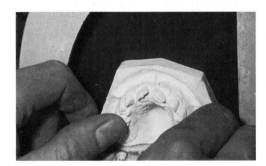

Figure D1.5 Trimming the base of the upper model to the scribed line

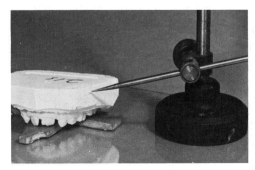

Figure D1.4 Scribing the upper model

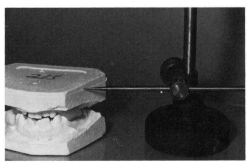

Figure D1.6 Scribing the base of the lower model. Note the size and position of the wax bite

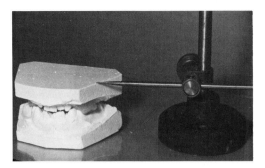

Figure D1.7 The lower model is cut to the correct depth. Note that the scribed line is still just visible

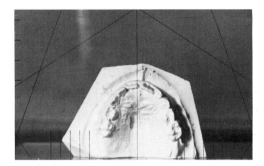

Figure D1.10 The upper model is cut with the back edge at right angles to the middle line of the palate. Note that the centre line of the dental arch does not in this case correspond with the middle line of the palate. The left upper lateral incisor is missing giving rise to an asymmetry

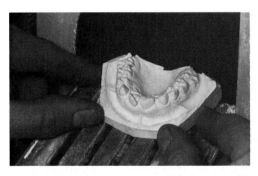

Figure D1.8 Cutting the back edge of the upper model

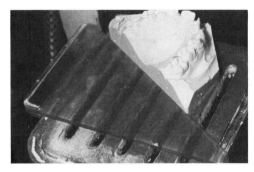

Figure D1.11 Trimming the front of the upper model. Right side

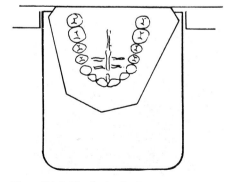

Figure D1.9 The back edge is trimmed at right angles to the middle line

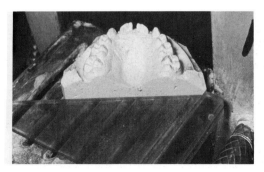

Figure D1.12 Trimming the front of the upper model. Left side

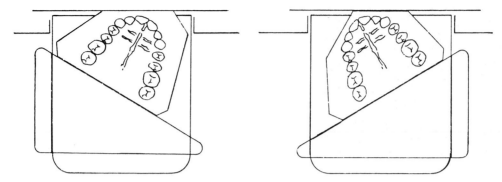

Figure D1.13 The front surfaces are cut so that the point is in line with the middle line of the palate

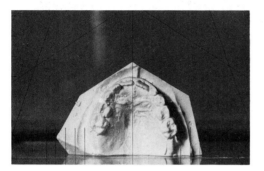

Figure D1.14 The point at the front of the model is in line with the centre line of the palate

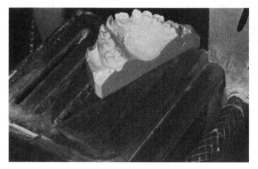

Figure D1.15 Trimming the left side of the model. The right side is similarly trimmed

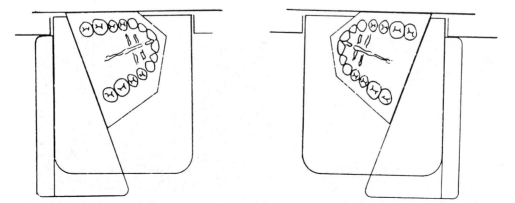

Figure D1.16 The sides of the model are cut symmetrically about the middle line

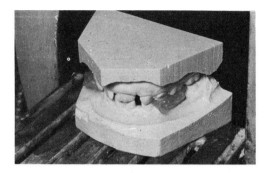

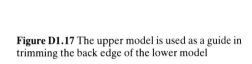

Figure D1.17 The upper model is used as a guide in trimming the back edge of the lower model

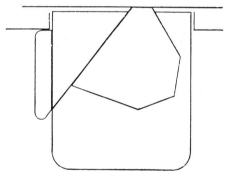

Figure D1.18 The upper model is used as a guide in trimming the sides of the lower model

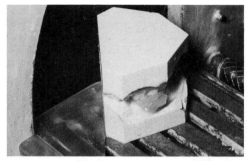

Figure D1.19 With the third set square the back corners of the upper and lower models are trimmed simultaneously

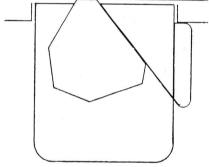

Figure D1.20 The distal corners are cut symmetrically to the middle line. This stage may conveniently be done with the models in occlusion

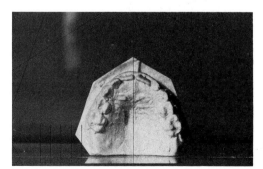

Figure D1.21 The upper model base is completely symmetrical

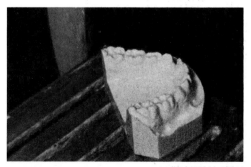

Figure D1.22 The front of the lower model is trimmed to a smooth curve

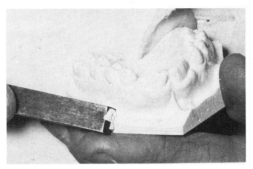

Figure D1.23 The rough edges are trimmed with a sharp chisel

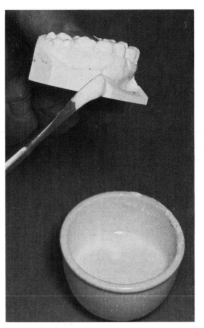

Figure D1.25 Air bubbles are filled with a smooth plaster mixture

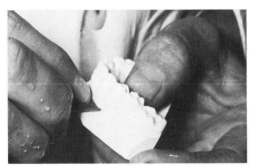

Figure D1.24 The curved cut edges are smoothed with wet-and-dry sandpaper

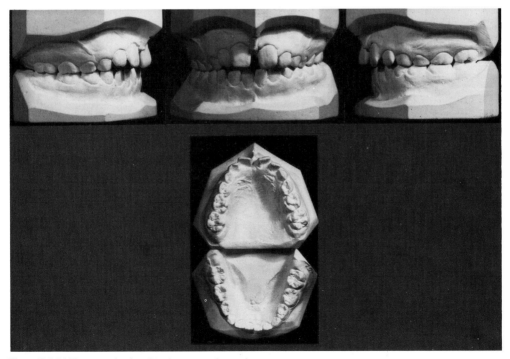

Figure D1.26 Photographs showing the casts to best advantage

It should be noted that the median palatal raphe is the only anatomical landmark visible on study casts. The upper cast is trimmed so as to be symmetrical about the median palatal raphe and not to the vertical line between the upper central incisors which may be asymmetrical. If the upper cast is trimmed to the centre line of the palate, any asymmetry of the upper incisors will be noticeable on looking at the record casts. The final effect is shown in *Figure D1.26.*

The casts should be dried in a warm place and the patient's name and number and date of record pencilled on the base. Casts should be stored in suitable boxes with a sheet of plastic foam 5 mm thick between the occlusal surfaces and an elastic band to keep the casts together (*Figure D1.27*).

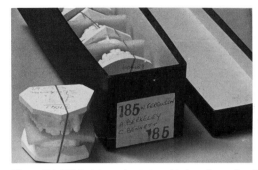

Figure D1.27 Models are best stored in long boxes 3 × 3 × 11 inches. Sheet plastic foam is put between the occlusal surfaces to protect the teeth

Appendix E

Materials for removable appliance construction

Stainless steel

Stainless steel as used in orthodontics is an alloy of iron containing nickel 18% and chromium 8%. Discovered, it is said, by accident when a batch of steel was 'contaminated' with chromium or nickel and thrown on the scrap heap where it did not rust, stainless steel was introduced for the construction of orthodontic appliances in Ireland by Friel (1933).

Stainless steel combines the properties of elasticity and malleability in good proportions so that wires of all gauges can be formed by appropriate bending methods and there is still adequate elasticity for springs.

The elasticity of this alloy is produced by the wire-drawing process which work-hardens the material as it is drawn through successively smaller dies and the hardness of the wire is expressed by the tensile strength as shown in *Table E1.1*. Wires

having tensile strengths shown in *Table E1.2* provide the most suitable properties for the construction of removable orthodontic appliances.

The choice of inches or millimetres for orthodontic materials depends on custom and upbringing but it is useful to know the equivalent gauges of wires in the two systems so that either may be used at will and dimensions transposed from one scale to the other when required. One metre equals 39.37 inches

Table E1.1 Conversion table for tensile strength*

Description	Tensile strength		
	lb/in² (USA)	tons/in²	kg/mm²
Hard or hard drawn	224 000–246 400	100–110	157–173
	246 400–268 800	110–120	173–189
	268 800–291 200	120–130	189–205
	291 200–313 600	130–140	205–220
	313 600–336 000	140–150	220–236
High tensile, spring hard, super hard	358 400 or more	160 or more	252 or more

Table E1.2 Tensile strength of stainless steel wires for orthodontic appliance construction*

Diameter (mm)	Tensile strength (tons/in²)	Application
1.5	100–110	Bows and arches
1.25		
1.0		
0.9	110–120	
0.8		
0.7		Clasps — Finger springs
0.6	120–130	Self-supporting springs
0.5		
0.4		
0.35	130–140	Springs supported on heavy arches
0.3		
0.25	140–150	Twin-wire arch — Coil springs
0.2		
0.15		
0.4		
0.45	160 or more	Arches for multiband appliances
0.5		
0.55		

* Extracts from British Standard 3507:1962, 'Specification for Orthodontic Wire and Tape and Dental Ligature Wire made of Stainless Steel' are reproduced by permission of the British Standards Institution, 2 Park Street, London W1, from whom copies of the complete standard may be purchased.

* Extracts from British Standard 3507:1962, 'Specification for Orthodontic Wire and Tape and Dental Ligature Wire made of Stainless Steel' are reproduced by permission of the British Standards Institution, 2 Park Street, London W1, from whom copies of the complete standard may be purchased.

and *Table E1.3* shows the equivalent values, suitably rounded, for wires commonly used in orthodontic practice.

Heat treatment of stainless steel wires

The bending of stainless steel wires produces work-hardening and sets up stresses which tend to return the wire to its original shape before bending.

In practice these effects on physical characteristics do not cause any problems in orthodontic appliance construction if care is taken not to overwork the wire and if necessary it is possible to relieve work stresses by controlled heating of the wire after it has been formed.

Stress-relief heat treatment can be achieved in archwires by heating with an electric current until the wire turns to a medium straw colour. Some orthodontic welders have terminals with a variable output of a few volts with which archwires can be treated (*Figure E1.1*). Complex archwires containing coils would not react uniformly to this method of heat treatment.

Another method, suitable for wires of any thickness and form, is to place the wires in an oven at an accurately controlled temperature of 399°C for ten minutes.

Table E1.3 Wire and tape thickness in millimetres and equivalent thickness in inches

mm	in	thousandth of an inch
1.5	0.059	60
1.25	0.049	50
1.0	0.039	40
0.9	0.035	36
0.8	0.032	32
0.7	0.028	28
0.65	0.026	26
0.6	0.024	24
0.55	0.022	22
0.5	0.020	20
0.45	0.018	18
0.4	0.016	16
0.35	0.014	14
0.3	0.012	12
0.25	0.010	10
0.2	0.008	8
0.15	0.006	6
0.1	0.004	4
0.05	0.002	2
0.025	0.001	1

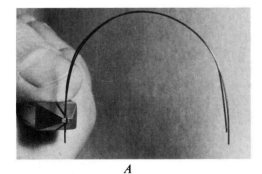

A

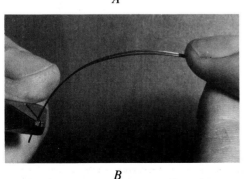

B

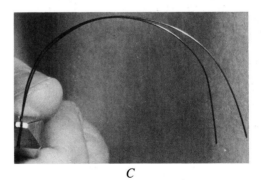

C

Figure E1.1 *A*, Two plain arches of 0.5 mm hard wire have been formed. One has been heat-treated, the other has not; *B*, the archwires are held side by side in strong pliers and stroked once or twice with a straightening movement of the fingers and thumb; *C*, the heat-treated wire has resisted the straightening effect to a marked degree; the untreated wire has shown a tendency to return to its original shape before it was bent into arch form

The acrylic resins

Heat-curing resins are still sometimes used for orthodontic appliances in which case it is necessary to construct the appliance in wax on a dental cast first of all.

After clasps and springs have been made, sheet wax is softened and pressed into place. Bite-planes are built up and the contours of the appliance developed and the outline trimmed. Only as much wax is added as is necessary for the functions of the appliance and for strength. In particular, a single thickness of wax is sufficient for the palate in upper appliances.

The waxed-up appliance is then invested in a flask, the wax washed out with boiling water and replaced with acrylic resin which is cured by boiling. This is a standard procedure for the production of appliances of various kinds in dentistry (*Figure E1.2*).

The use of cold- or self-curing acrylic resin speeds the production and repair of removable orthodontic appliances and this material has largely replaced heat-curing resin.

The wire work of appliances is constructed as usual but the wax used to attach these parts to the working cast is disposed so as to hold the wires and cover those areas where the acrylic material is not

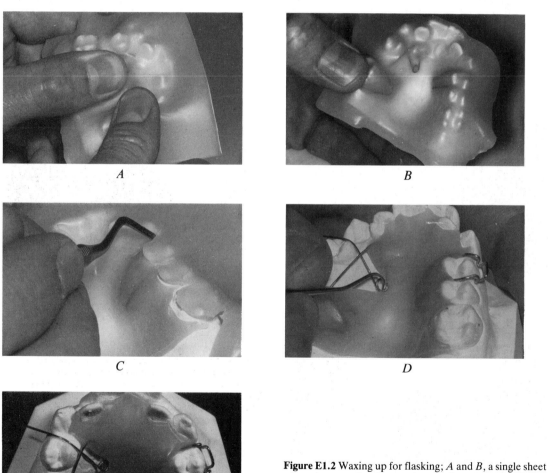

A

B

C

D

E

Figure E1.2 Waxing up for flasking; *A* and *B*, a single sheet of wax is warmed and pressed evenly into contact with the moistened model. The wax is flamed again around the teeth and pressed firmly into contact with the plaster; *C*, the wax is trimmed accurately to shape with a single cut with a double flat-ended plastic instrument; *D* and *E*, the edges of the wax are flamed again and pressed firmly down on to the model and any wax inside or about the coils of springs is removed with a probe

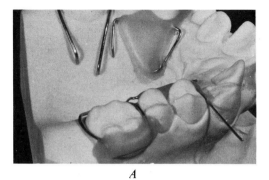

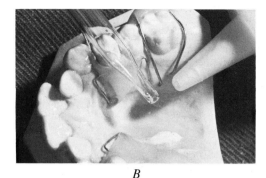

A	*B*

Figure E1.3 *A*, Clasps and springs are attached to the model with pink wax. For the springs, the pink wax serves to block out areas which do not need to be reproduced in acrylic material and also holds the wires in place; *B*, liquid is dropped on with a dropper and the powder blown on from a soft polythene bottle. Note that the position of the model controls the flow of the acrylic mixture. One side of an appliance should be completed and have begun to set before the other is commenced. For the construction of the front part of the baseplate, the model is placed with the incisors downwards

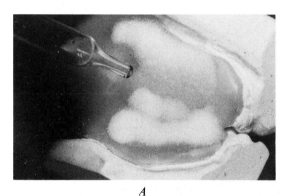

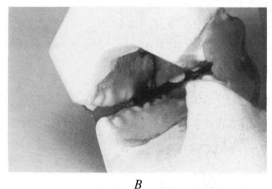

A	*B*

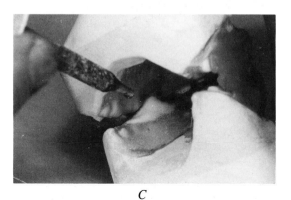

C

Figure E1.4 *A*, Using cold-curing acrylic resin to build up an oral screen after a layer of wax has been moulded over the working casts to give the necessary distancing of the screen from the soft tissues; *B*, the construction of the Andresen appliance in cold-curing resin. The upper and lower components are made separately and then while still on the articulated working casts, are joined at three points with small amounts of resin to ensure their correct relationship. (The patch of resin in the left buccal segments has been darkened to make it slightly more visible.) These small amounts of resin are allowed to polymerize. The casts are removed from the articulator and the bases cut down to allow the whole workpiece to go into the hydro-flask; *C*, the bulk of the resin to join the halves is then added, a layer of wax applied to the outside controlling the flow of the resin. The new mass of resin is cured in a pressure flask so avoiding porosity. The complete appliance is trimmed and polished in the usual way

required. After the cast has been coated with a separating medium the resin is then built up by puffing on powdered resin and dropping the monomer onto the powder. The cast must be turned in different directions to control the build up of the resin and when the baseplate is satisfactorily contoured, polymerization is completed in warm water under pressure. The whole operation can be done more quickly than by waxing up and using heat-curing material (*Figure E1.3*).

The oral screen and Andresen appliance can also be made in cold-curing acrylic resin as the construction does not take as long as waxing up and using heat-curing material.

To construct the oral screen, the working casts are covered with a layer of pink wax to give the necessary clearance between the finished screen and the soft tissues. The wax is scraped away at points where the screen is to make contact with the teeth.

The acrylic resin is applied by puffing on from a soft plastic bottle and dropping monomer to bind the powder together (*Figure E1.4A*). When the area of the screen has been covered, the resin is cured in a pressure flask, removed from the casts, trimmed and polished. The material is, of course, a clear resin.

The Andresen appliance is made by constructing the upper and lower parts separately in cold-curing resin and then joining the two together. As the joining process takes a considerable thickness of resin with the attendant risk of porosity, the parts are, therefore, first joined at three points with small quantities of resin which is allowed to cure spontaneously, which occurs in 20 to 30 minutes at room temperature (*Figure E1.4B*).

The casts are then removed from the articulator and cut down so that the whole workpiece will go into a pressure flask. The space between the upper and lower parts is then filled in with resin and cured in a pressure flask without any risk of the registration of the working bite being disturbed (*Figure E1.4C*). After curing, the appliance is removed from the casts and trimmed and polished in the usual way.

Appendix F

An orthodontic coil spring winder

Coil springs have various uses in removable and fixed appliance techniques and, although coil springs are available from orthodontic suppliers, the spring winder described here is intended to allow the user to produce springs of the exact size and strength he requires.

A winder like this was described by Porter (1941, 1943) and a variation was introduced to the Eastman Dental Hospital, London by Mr J. S. Beresford. The design illustrated was conceived as offering optimum strength and speed in operation but the underlying principle is not different from the earlier models.

The winding jig consists of a length of 1.0 mm internal stainless steel tube and a short length of 0.5 mm internal stainless steel tube fixed at right angles. These are soldered to adjacent edges of a plate of stainless steel sheet.

The springs are wound on mandrels of stainless steel wire from 0.5 mm to 1.0 mm in thickness soldered into the shafts of mandrels such as are used for polishing discs. A small diaphragm with a fine hole in it is soldered at the root of the mandrel. The spring wire is held in this hole for winding and the completed spring is easily removed from this attachment when tension is released (*Figures F1.1–F1.6*).

When winding springs it is important to rotate the mandrel slowly so that the mandrel can be withdrawn smoothly from the tube and the spring coils made to lie close together, especially if fine wire is being coiled. This means that an engine with a slow speed must be available. Care must be taken not to let the coils overlap and build up and jam the winder or to allow the free end of the wire to become looped around a finger.

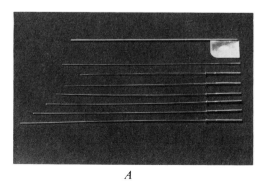
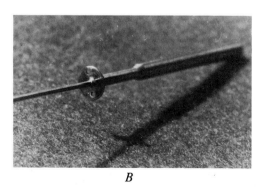

A *B*

Figure F1.1 *A*, Winding jig, lining tube and six winding mandrels sizes 1.0, 0.9, 0.8, 0.7, 0.6 and 0.5 mm thick. The mandrels are graduated in length from thickest to thinnest, so that selection of the required size is facilitated; *B*, a mandrel showing the shank, made from a bur or straight handpiece mandrel with a disc 5–6 mm diameter and perforated in two places. One of these holes is used to retain the spring wire during winding of the spring

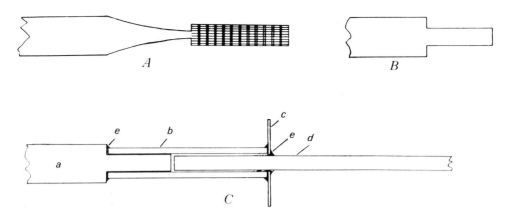

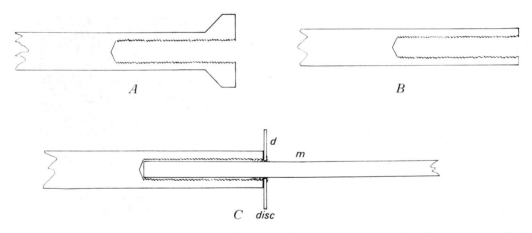

Figure F1.2 Construction of winding mandrel from a straight handpiece bur shank; *A*, bur, any kind can be used; *B*, bur ground down forming stub 3–5 mm long and 1.0 mm thick; *C*, 1.0 mm tubing soldered over stub. A long piece is used to facilitate soldering and the tubing is then cut off leaving 1.0 cm attached to the bur (*a*, *b*). The winding wire *d* is then fitted in and a plate of steel tape, *c*, is fitted over the wire and the whole soldered together at *e*

Figure F1.3 *A*, Construction of a winding mandrel from a straight handpiece mandrel; *B*, the flange is ground off; *C*, the plate of stainless steel, *d*, and winding wire, *m*, are fitted as in *Figure F1.2* and soldered together

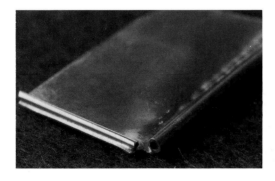

Figure F1.4 The relationship of the working ends of the winding tube, 1.0 mm in diameter, and the feeder tube, 0.5 mm in diameter

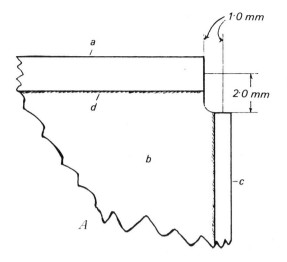

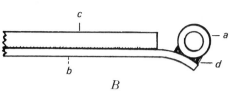

Figure F1.5 *A*, Plan of the arrangement of the ends of the winder and feeder tubes. The dimensions shown should be carefully observed to secure the best results; *B*, view of the winding tube, end on. Note that the edge of the tube is level with the centre of the winding tube. It is then possible to wind springs in either direction with equal tension. *a*, main or winding tube; *b*, steel baseplate material; *c*, feeder tube; *d*, solder

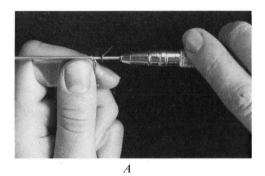

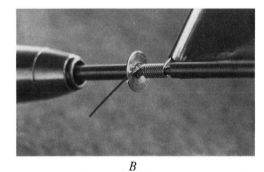

Figure F1.6 *A*, The winder in use. The spring wire is controlled by the fingers of the left hand. The wire can be seen entering from below. A slow winding speed should be used; *B*, the winder in use. This spring is being wound in a right-handed manner. The mandrel may, however, be equally well rotated in the opposite direction

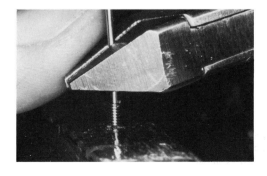

Figure F1.7 Pressing an archwire into a friction-fit stop. The archwire is tapered slightly at the end and is held in Adams Universal Pliers near to the end of the arch. The end of the archwire is placed in the stop which is rested on a piece of soft wood. Using the thumb of the other hand on the pliers beaks, the archwire is pressed into and through the stop

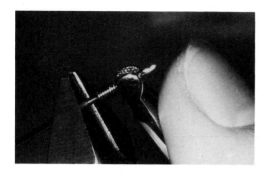

Figure F1.8 Positioning the friction-fit stop on the archwire. The archwire is gripped in Adams Universal Pliers using the left hand. The stop is a short way from the pliers. This distance can be predetermined so making accurate movement of the stop very easy. Note the tapering end of the 1.0 mm archwire. Howe pliers are placed over the projecting end of the archwire which is held lightly using the right hand. The left thumb is placed on top of the Howe pliers and the stop is pressed along the archwire until it comes up against the Universal Pliers

Coil springs to be used in compression are made by stretching a closely wound spring while still on its mandrel and compressing it again. The spring will remain expanded and can then be used in compression.

Friction-fit stops for heavy archwires are made from 0.35 mm hard wire wound on a mandrel 0.1 mm smaller than the archwire. Five or six coils of the spring are pressed onto the archwire after slightly rounding or tapering the end and, holding the archwire with Universal Pliers, the stop may be adjusted for position by pressing along the arch using Howe pliers (*Figures F1.7* and *F1.8*).

Bibliography

Adams C. P. (1950) A method for teaching the fundamentals of wire bending technique. *Trans. Br. Soc. Study Orthod.* 71–75.

Adams C. P. (1955) *The Design and Construction of Removable Orthodontic Appliances,* 1st Edition, John Wright and Sons Ltd, Bristol.

Adams C. P. (1969) An investigation into indications for and the effects of the function regulator. *Trans. Eur. Orthod. Soc.* 293–312.

Adams C. P. (1983) Letter to the Editor. *Br. J. Orthod.* **10**, 167.

Andresen V. (1936) The Norwegian system of functional gnatho-orthopaedics. *Acta Gnath. Kbh.* **1**, No. 1.

Andrews L. F. (1972) The six keys to normal occlusion. *Am. J. Orthod.* **63**, 296.

Angle E. H. (1903–4) A masterpiece. (The sin of extraction for regulation purposes). *Commonwealth Dent. Rev.* **I**, 26.

Angle E. H. (1907) *Treatment of Malocclusion of the Teeth.* The S.S. White Dental Manufacturing Company, Philadelphia.

Angle E. H. (1910) Bone growing: a problem in orthodontic treatment. *Dent. Cosmos* **LII**, 261–267.

Angle E. H. (1929) The latest and best in orthodontic mechanism. *Dent. Cosmos* **70**, 1143–1158; **71**, 164–175, 260–270.

Backofen W. A. and Gales G. F. (1951) The low temperature heat treatment of stainless steel. *Angle Orthod.* **21**, 117–124.

Backofen W. A. and Gales G. F. (1952) Heat treating stainless steel for orthodontics. *Am. J. Orthod.* **38**, 755–765.

Badcock J. H. (1911) The screw expansion plate. *Trans. Br. Soc. Study Orthod.* **3**, 3–8.

Baker, H. A. (1904) Treatment of protruding and receding jaws by the use of inter-maxillary elastics. *Int. Dent. J.* **25**, 344–356.

Balters W. (1952) Hendernisse und Hemmungen bei der Kieferdehnung. In Korkhaus G. (ed.) *Die Kiefererweiterung, Moglichkeiten und Grenzun. Zahn-, Mund- und Kieferheilkunde in Vortragen,* Heft 7, pp. 100–105, Munchen, Carl Hanser Verlag.

Balters W. (1965) Die Technik und Ubung der allgemeinen und speziellen Bionator-Therapie. *Quintessence* **5**, 77–85.

Balters W. (1973) *Ein Einfuhrung in die Bionator-heilmethode; ausgewahlte Schriften und Vortrage,* Heidelberg, C. Herrmann.

Bass N. M. (1975) Early treatment of skeletal II malocclusion involving preliminary incisor root torquing. *Trans. Eur. Orthod. Soc.* 191–200.

Begg P. R. (1965) *Begg Orthodontic Theory and Technique,* Philadelphia, W. B. Saunders (3rd edition, 1977, edited by Begg P. R. and Kesling P. C.).

Bell R. D. (1932) Electric resistance spot welding. *Dent. Rec.* **52**, 554–566.

Charlier M. (1928) La technique des alliages inoxydables et celle de leur sourdure electrique. *Odontologie.* **67**, 645–651.

Clark W. J. (1982) The twin block traction technique. *Eur. J. Orthod.* **4**, 130–138.

Clemmer E. J. and Hayes E. W. (1979) Patient cooperation in wearing orthodontic headgear. *Am. J. Orthod.* **75**, 517–524.

Coffin W. H. (1881) A generalized treatment of irregularities. *Trans. Int. Congr. Med.,* 7th Session, London, Vol. III, 542–547.

de Coster L. (1931a) Une technique systematique d'appareillage orthodontique en acier inoxydable. *Province Dentaire,* **17**, 201–222.

de Coster L. (1931b) The use of rustless steel in dentofacial orthopaedics. *Int. Orthod. Congr.* **2**, 475–479; also in *Int. J. Orthod.* (1932) **18**, 1191–1195.

Cousins A. J. P. (1962) Removable appliance technique: the application of rapid cold-cure acrylic resin. *Dent. Practit.* **13**, 29–32.

193

Crozat G. B. (1920) Possibilities and use of removable labiolingual spring appliances. *Int. J. Orthodontia.* **6**, 1–7.

Cutler R. (1932) A new preparation of British stainless steel. *Trans. Br. Soc. Study Orthod.* 1–15.

Duyzings J. A. C. (1954) *Orthodontische Apparatur,* Amsterdam, Dental-Depot A. M. Disselkoen, pp. 33, 35 and 37.

Eckert-Möbius A. (1953) Normale and pathologische Physiologie der Nasen and Mandatmang. *Dtsch. Zahn-, Mund- u. Kieferheilk.* **18**, 346–378.

Eckert-Möbius A. (1962) Grenzprobleme der Zahn-Mund- and Kieferheilkunde und der Hals-, Nasen- und Ohrenheilkunde aus rhinologischer Sicht. *Dtsch. Zahn-, Mund- u. Kieferheilk.* **37**, 216–225.

Eckert-Möbius A. (1963) Grundsatzliches zur Atmung als rhinologisch-kieferorthopadisches Problem. *Acta Otolaryngol. (Stockh.) Suppl.* **183**, 36–38.

Endicott C. L., Pedley V. G. and Grossmann W. (1947) Practical and theoretical observations on the Norwegian system. *Trans. Br. Soc. Study. Orthod.* 31–60.

Enlow D. H., Moyers R. E., Hunter W. S. and McNamara J. A. (1969) A procedure for the analysis of intrinsic facial form and growth. *Am. J. Orthod.* **56**, 6–23.

Fränkel R. (1964) Luftdruck, Atmung und die orofazialen Weichteile. *Dtsch. Zahn-, Mund- u. Kieferheilk.* **43**, 367–374.

Fränkel R. (1966) The theoretical concept underlying treatment with function correctors. *Trans. Eur. Orthod. Soc.* 233–250.

Fränkel R. (1966) *Funktionskieferothopadie und der Mundvorhof als apparative Basis,* Berlin, Verlag Volk und Gesundheit.

Friel E. S. (1933) The practical application of stainless steel in the construction of fixed orthodontic appliances. *Trans. Br. Soc. Study Orthod.* 23.

Friel E. S. and McKeag H. T. A. (1939) The design and construction of fixed orthodontic appliances in stainless steel. *Dent. Rec.* **59**, 359–390; also *Trans. Eur. Orthod. Soc.* (1938) **22**, 53–84.

Funk A. C. (1951) The heat treatment of stainless steel. *Angle Orthod.* **21**, 129–138.

Graber T. M. and Neumann, B. (1984) *Removable Orthodontic Appliances,* 2nd Edition, W. B. Saunders and Company.

Grude R. (1938) The Norwegian system of orthodontic treatment. *Dent. Rec.* **58**, 529–551.

Hallett G. E. M. (1952) Cold curing acrylic resin as an aid in orthodontics. *Br. Dent. J.* **92**, 294–295.

Harvold E. P. (1974) *The Activator in Interceptive Orthodontics,* St. Louis, C. V. Mosby.

Harvold E. P. and Vargervik K. (1971) Morphogenetic response to activator treatment. *Am. J. Orthod.* **60**, 478–479.

Haupl K., Grossmann W. I. and Clarkson P. (1952) *Textbook of Functional Jaw Orthopaedics,* London, Kimpton.

Hawley C. A. (1925) Principles and art of retention. *Int. J. Orthod.* **xi**, 315.

Hawley C. A. (1919) A removable retainer. *Int. J. Orthod. Oral Surg.* **2**, 291–298.

Haynes S. (1982) Discontinuation of orthodontic treatment in the General Dental Service in England and Wales 1972–1979. *Br. Dent. J.* **152**, 127–129.

Hill C. V. (1954) Controlled tooth movement. Multiband round arch technique. *Dent. Practit.* **5**, 2–13, 52–63.

Hopkin G. B. (1958) The rubber peg plate. *Trans. Br. Soc. Study Orthod.* 86–87; also *Dent. Practit.* (1958) **9**, 86–87.

Hoyle A. (1983) The development of removable appliances in the United Kingdom. *Br. J. Orthod.* **10**, 73–77.

Jackson V. H. (1904) *Orthodontia and Orthopedia of the Face,* Philadelphia, J. B. Lippincott.

Jackson V. H. (1906) Orthodontia. *Dent. Cosmos,* **48**, 278–284.

Johnson I. E. (1938) The twin-wire appliance. *Am. J. Orthod.* **24**, 300–327.

Johnson I. E. (1941) The construction and manipulation of the twin-wire arch mechanism. *Am. J. Orthod.* **27**, 289–307.

Johnson W. T. (1952) A friction fit attachment. *Trans. Br. Soc. Study Orthod.* 65–69; also *Dent. Rec.* (1953) **73**, 326–330.

Kerr W. J. S. (1984) Appliance breakages. *Br. J. Orthod.* **11**, 137–142.

Kerr W. J. S. and TenHave T. R. (1988) A comparison of three appliance systems in the treatment of Class III malocclusions. *Eur. J. Orthod.* **10**, 269–280.

Kerr W. J. S., TenHave T. R. and McNamara J. A. (1989) A comparison of skeletal and dental changes produced by function regulators (F.R.2 and F.R.3). *Eur. J. Orthod.* **11**, 235–242.

Kesling H. D. (1945) The philosophy of the tooth positioning appliance. *Am. J. Orthod.* **31**, 297–304.

Korbitz A. (1914) *Kursus der systematischen Orthodontik,* 2nd Edition, Leipzig, Verlag H. Licht.

Korkhaus G. (1960) Present orthodontic thought in Germany. Experiences with the Norwegian method of functional orthopaedics in the treatment of distocclusion. *Am. J. Orthod.* **46**, 270–287.

Leech H. L. (1951) Appliances in the treatment of the collapsed lower arch. *Trans. Br. Soc. Study Orthod.* 94–98.

McCallin S. G. (1954) Retraction of maxillary teeth with removable appliances using intermaxillary or extra-oral traction. *Dent. Rec.* **74**, 36–41.

McCoy I. D. (1941) *Applied Orthodontics,* London, Kimpton.

McKeag H. T. A. (1921) Orthodontic education. *Trans. Br. Soc. Orthod.* 9–13.

McKeag H. T. A. (1928) Physical laws and the design of orthodontic appliances. *Trans. Br. Soc. Study Orthod.* 69–87.

McKeag H. T. A. (1935) The teaching of appliance design in orthodontia. *Trans. Br. Soc. Study Orthod.* 260–277.

McNamara J. A., Bookstein F. L. and Shaughnessy T. G. (1985) Skeletal and dental changes following function regulator therapy on Class II patients. *Am. J. Orthod.* **88**, 91–110.

Moss M. L. (1962) Cephalometric changes during functional appliance therapy. *Trans. Eur. Orthod. Soc.* 327–341.

Nolteimier H. (1949) *Eirfuhrung in die allgemeine Kezfer- und Gesichtsorthopadie*, Vols. I, II, Alfeld, Buchdruckerei P. Dobler.

Oliver O. A., Irish R. E. and Wood C. R. (1940) *Labiolingual Technique*, London, Kimpton.

Packham A. L. (1932) In Discussion on paper by Cutler R. (see above).

Parfitt G. I. and Friel E. S. (1946) Experimental welder design. *Trans. Br. Soc. Study Orthod.* 105–120; also *Dent. Rec.* (1947) **67**, 250–259.

Porter L. I. (1941) Johnson twin arch technique. *Am. J. Orthod.* **27**, 577–583.

Porter L. I. (1943) Johnson twin arch technique and special arch pulling vice. *Am. J. Orthod.* **29**, 348–354.

Reitan K. (1985) Biomechanical principles and reactions. In Graber T. M. and Swain B. F. (eds) *Orthodontics: Current Principles and Techniques*, St Louis, C. V. Mosby.

Richardson A. and Adams C. P. (1963) An investigation into the short and long term effects of the anterior bite-plane on the occlusal relationship and facial form. *Trans. Eur. Orthod. Soc.* 375–383.

Riolo M. L., Moyers R. E., McNamara J. A. Jnr and Hunter W. S. (1974) *An Atlas of Craniofacial Growth. Monograph 2. Craniofacial Growth Series*, pp. 355–356, University of Michigan Press.

Roberts G. H. (1956) A removable incisor retractor. *Dent. Practit.* **7**, 220–221.

Robin P. (1902) Demonstration pratique sur la construction et la mise en bouche d'un nouvel appareil de redressement. *Rev. Stomatol.*, Paris, **9**, 561–590.

Rossi E. B. (1954) *Welding Engineering*, New York, McGraw-Hill.

Roux W. (1895) *Funktionelle Anpassung. Realencyclopaedie der gesamten Heilkunde, Bd. 8*, Vienna, Eulenberg.

Schwarz A. M. (1932) Tissue changes incidental to orthodontic tooth movement. *Int. J. Orthod., Oral Surg. Radiol.*, **18**, 331–352.

Schwarz A. M. (1933) Tissue changes incidental to orthodontic tooth movement. *2nd Int. Orthod. Congr.* pp. 123–244. St. Louis, C. V. Mosby.

Schwarz A. M. (1954) *Die Zahn-, Mund- und Kieferheilkunde.* pp. 450–457, Munich, Urban.

Schwarz A. M. (1956) *Lehrgand der Gebissregelung, Bd II*, Munich, Urban.

Simon P. (1926) On the necessity of gnathostatic diagnosis in orthodontic practice. *Int. J. Orthod.* **12**, 1102–1113.

Softley I. W (1953) Cephalometric changes in seven 'post-normal' cases treated by the Andresen method. *Dent. Rec.* **73**, 485–494.

Strang R. H. W. (1950) *A Textbook of Orthodontia*, London, Kimpton.

Sved A. (1944) Changing the occlusal level and a new method of retention. *Am. J. Orthod. Oral Surg.* **30**, 527–535.

Watkin H. G. (1933) Treated cases. *Trans. Br. Soc. Study Orthod.* 30.

Watry F. M. (1947) A contribution to the history of physiotherapeutics in maxillofacial orthopedics. *Trans. Eur. Orthod. Soc.* 56–63.

White T. C., Gardiner J. H. and Leighton B. C. (1954) *Orthodontics for Dental Students*, London, Staples, (3rd edition, 1976, London, Macmillan).

Wild N. (1950) Design and behaviour of orthodontic springs. *Trans. Br. Soc. Study Orthod.* 109–120.

Wilson H. E. (1953) Myofunctional appliances. *Dent. Practit.* **4**, 70–78.

Woolass K. F., Shaw W. C., Viader P. H. and Lewis A. S. (1988) The prediction of patient cooperation in orthodontic treatment. *Eur. J. Orthod.* **10**, 235–243.

Index